Chen Tuan's
Four Season Internal Kungfu

Chen Tuan's
Four Season Internal Kungfu

Breathing Methods, Exercises,
Herbs and Foods for Longevity

Translation and Commentary
by Stuart Alve Olson

Edited by Patrick D. Gross

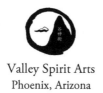

Valley Spirit Arts
Phoenix, Arizona

Disclaimer

Please note that the author and publisher of this work are not responsible for any injury that may result from practicing the techniques or following the instructions given within. Since some of the physical activities described in this book may be too strenuous in nature for some readers to engage in safely, it is advised that a physician be consulted before training.

Note: The preferred Pinyin spellings of Chinese terms is used throughout the book except in the spellings of *Tao* (Dao) and *Kung* (Gong). Spelling Tao with a "T" instead of a "D" is more common and recognizable in English, likewise "Kung," as in *Kungfu,* is more common as well.

Copyright © 2016 by Stuart Alve Olson.

All rights reserved. No part of this book may be reproduced or used in any form or by any means, electronic or mechanical, including photocopying, recording, or by any information storage and retrieval system, without prior written permission from Stuart Alve Olson and Valley Spirit Arts.

Library of Congress Control Number: 2016940616
ISBN-13: 978-1-5330-5010-6

Valley Spirit Arts, LLC
www.valleyspiritarts.com
contact@valleyspiritarts.com

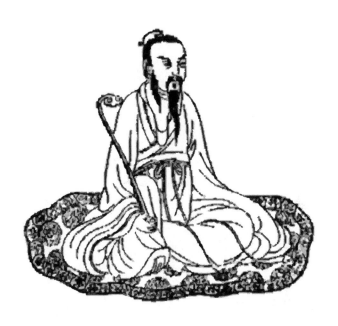

太極尺始創者陳摶老祖畫像

An Authentic Image of the Venerable Founder
and Creator of Taiji Ruler, Chen Tuan

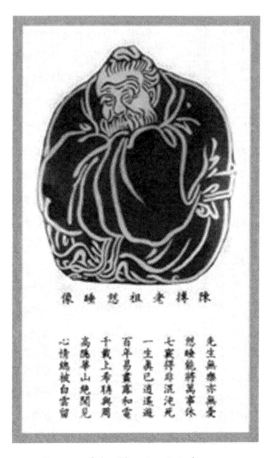

Image of the Sleeping Meditator,
Venerable Ancestor Chen Tuan

Acknowledgments

"Teaching is the best teacher."
—Master T.T. Liang

To my teacher, Master T.T. Liang, for opening the door to this incredible world of internal alchemy.

Much appreciation to Patrick Gross for all his efforts in making this book.

To all my students, past and present, for their questions, support, and encouragement on this path of inner discovery.

I bow in deepest gratitude to all.

Contents

Preface xiii
About Chen Tuan xix
Introduction 1
Chen Tuan's Two Yearly Regimes 5
The Six Zi and Classifications of Qi Influences 11
Six Zi and The Twelve Primary Qi Meridians 25
    Ultimate Yang Meridians 28
    Ultimate Yin Meridians 32
    Young Yang Meridians 36
    Young Yin Meridians 40
    Bright Yang Meridians 44
    Faint Yin Meridians 48
    The Control and Function Meridians 52
The Internal Organs and Functions 57
    Five Viscera 57
    Six Bowels 58
Elemental Activities 63
    The Six Zi Responding with the Six Qi Diagram ... 65
    Secondary Fire 67
Use of Herbs and Foods 71
Preliminary Instructions 75
    Breathing Methods and Regimes 75
    Breathing Patterns in the Exercises 80
    Massaging Qi Centers and Meridians 81
    Daily Practice Advice 83

Spring

Spring Kung 87
    Green Dragon Kung 93
    Herbs for Cleansing and Nourishing the Liver 97
    Foods for Expelling Foul Airs (Detoxing) of the Liver 98
The Six Dao Yin Seated Exercises of Spring 99
    First Spring Exercise 99
    Second Spring Exercise 105
    Third Spring Exercise 111
    Fourth Spring Exercise 117
    Fifth Spring Exercise 123
    Sixth Spring Exercise 127

Summer

Summer Kung 133
    Red Bird Kung 137
    Herbs for Nourishing the Heart 142
    Foods for Expelling Foul Airs (Detoxing) of the Heart ... 143
The Six Dao Yin Seated Exercises of Summer 145
    First Summer Exercise 145
    Second Summer Exercise 151
    Third Summer Exercise 155
    Fourth Summer Exercise 161
    Fifth Summer Exercise 167
    Sixth Summer Exercise 171
Late Summer and Long Summer Exercises 175

Autumn

Autumn Kung 179
    White Tiger Kung 183
    Herbs for Cleansing and Nourishing the Lungs 186
    Foods for Expelling Foul Airs (Detoxing) of the Lungs ... 187
Six Dao Yin Seated Exercises for Autumn 189
    First Autumn Exercise 189
    Second Autumn Exercise 195
    Third Autumn Exercise 201
    Fourth Autumn Exercise 205
    Fifth Autumn Exercise 209
    Sixth Autumn Exercise 213

Winter

Winter Kung 219
    Black Tortoise Kung 223
    Herbs for Cleansing and Nourishing the Kidneys 226
    Foods for Expelling Foul Airs (Detoxing)
        of the Kidneys 227
Six Dao Yin Seated Exercises for Winter 229
    First Winter Exercise 229
    Second Winter Exercise 235
    Third Winter Exercise 241
    Fourth Winter Exercise 247
    Fifth Winter Exercise 253
    Sixth Winter Exercise 259

Taoist Supine Methods

Chen Tuan Two Supine Methods 265
    Lying on the Right Side Kung 267
    Chen Xiyi's Lying on the Left Side Kung 273
Other Supine Methods 277
    Taoist Priestess Huang Hua's Sleeping on Ice Pose 277
    Yin Qinghe's Sleeping Method 278
    Celestial Master Xu Jing's Sleeping Kung 279
    Chen's Natural Attainment of the
        Great Sleeping Kung 280

Medicinal Kung Regimes

The Venerable Sovereign Li Playing the Lute Pose 285
    Exercise 286
    Herbal Formula 286
    Verses 287
Xu Shenweng's Method for Preserving the Qi
    and Opening the Passes 291
    Exercise 293
    Verse on Death 294
    Herbal Formula 295
    Verses 295

Appendix

Correlations and Positions of the Meridians
    According to the Eight Diagrams and Nine Palaces 301
Twelve Earthly Branches 310
Six Zi Calculations and *Yi Jing* Associations 312
Chart of the Five Forces Correlations 314
About the Translator 317

Preface

The Nourishing Life Arts (養生術, Yang Sheng Shu)[1] of Taoism are divided into two categories of practice: *External Elixir* (外丹, Waidan) and *Internal Elixir* (內丹, Neidan). Waidan practices not only help bring about optimum health and longevity, but they also serve as the foundational processes and precursors for the cultivation of Neidan. The goal of Neidan is the attainment of either physical or spiritual immortality through a transformational process of awakening, or returning to, the innate forces lying dormant within a person.

In Taoism, the meaning of "elixir," a term adapted by the Chinese alchemist of antiquity, is defined as a metallurgical medicinal compound for the cure of aging, illness, and death. Early Taoist alchemists believed that turning base metals into potable gold (the elixir) was the answer for the cessation of mortal conditions. They professed that the forging of base metals (white lead, black lead, mercury, and cinnabar, for example), along with specific protocols for the use of a furnace and cauldron, would produce a compound that could then be further

---

[1] *Nourishing Life Arts* (養生術, Yang Sheng Shu) is a broad term, encompassing everything from acupuncture and herbs to practices like Taijiquan, Eight Brocades, meditation, and Waidan and Neidan exercises. Basically, it's an umbrella term for all the Chinese arts directed at health, longevity, and immortality.

refined into potable gold, granting immortality to those who succeeded in the refinement process of making it and then imbibing this potable gold.

The idea of the *forging process* later became identified with creating the External Elixir (granting optimum health and longevity), and the *refinement process* became associated with forming the Internal Elixir (granting immortality).

The ingredients of lead, mercury, and cinnabar (as well as numerous other mineral composites) were later viewed as covert code for the physical and spiritual energies—specifically, the Three Treasures of Essence (精, Jing), Vitality/Breath (氣, Qi), and Spirit (神, Shen)—which form the External and Internal elixirs.

Likewise, this *forging* of Jing, Qi, and Shen (which Taoism refers to as *Setting Up the Foundation* or as *Replenishing the Three Treasures),* is the purpose and process of Waidan practices. The *refinement* of the Three Treasures (referred to as *Reverting* or *Transmuting the Elixir)* is the purpose and process of Neidan practices.

The exercise regimes contained within this work fall under the category of Waidan, as they are a most effective and expedient gateway to the Neidan process.

Waidan translates as External Elixir. *External* refers to the energies of the body you already have and can sense through the seasonal exercises presented in this work, but also from practices like acupuncture and through many other arts such as Taijiquan, Qigong, and so on. The meaning of "elixir" in the case of External Elixir (Waidan) practice is basically the experience of Qi from the movement and opening of the Qi meridians and cavities (Qi points) that readily operate in the body.

Whether or not you do any of these practices, everyone (and every living thing) has Qi meridians and cavities. Chinese medicine and herbal practices are based on working with these meridians and cavities for both the prevention and healing of illnesses, so the meaning of the term "elixir" is more like saying a medicine, a medicine of our own inherent system of Qi.

The purpose of Waidan (or Medical Qigong as it is now being presented) is to open all our meridians and Qi points so they can function properly, as well as to strengthen and preserve our Five Viscera (Organs), Six Bowels, blood and Qi circulatory systems, and the muscular system, from which we gain good health and longevity. Thus, the External Elixir is like "an external medicine" that heals our physical functions.

Neidan, translating as Internal Elixir, is a different system with its goal of attaining immortality. Granted, there's a great deal of overlap between the two ideas of External Elixir and Internal Elixir, as some meridians and Qi points share the same names and External Elixir practices are, for the most part, a precursor to taking on Internal Alchemy. The difference is that in External Alchemy the energies being dealt with are already there and just need stimulation to make use of and feel. In Internal Alchemy, the "elixir" is not present. It dried up slowly after our umbilical cord was severed.

We had this elixir when in our mother's womb, which aided our development during the gestation period. Once a person enters this world, however, the elixir diminishes and dries up. All that remains is our Original Spirit (元神, Yuan Shen), which lies hidden and obscured within our lower Elixir Field (丹田, Dan Tian, lower abdomen), another residual effect of the umbilical cord being cut. We breathe differently from when we were in the womb, and we experience senses that were non-existent in the womb. The task of Internal Alchemy is the recall of not only the elixir that ran freely through our body when in the womb, but also the functioning of our Original Spirit. Neither the elixir nor Original Spirit can functionally exist until we cultivate their return.

In analogy, Waidan is like the caterpillar, while Neidan is the butterfly. The purpose of this book then is the work of the caterpillar forming its cocoon—more precisely what Taoism calls *Setting Up the Foundation* for the practice of Internal Alchemy. Applying the teachings in *Refining the Elixir* are what lead to the metamorphosis of the caterpillar turning into a butterfly, as that book focuses on Internal Alchemy.

My intent for compiling this book was not to just present Chen Tuan's Dao Yin methods, but rather to show how intrinsically connected the teachings of External Alchemy are with those of Internal Alchemy. So in many ways this work is a companion volume to my book *Refining the Elixir*. This book serves as a bridge between Waidan and

Neidan or, in another view, it is directed at the After Heaven processes, while *Refining the Elixir* goes more to the Before Heaven processes. A serious cultivator needs to study and pursue both theory and practice of External and Internal Alchemy.

As the *Jade Tablet Decrees on Nature and Life* (性命圭旨, *Xing Ming Gui Zhi*) and other great Taoist alchemy books state, "Use the After Heaven to enter the Before Heaven." More simply put, you need to construct a cocoon if you ever hope to become a butterfly, and this work is focused on learning how to build that cocoon.

About Chen Tuan

陳 搏

The creation of these exercises are attributed to the famous Taoist adept and immortal sage Chen Tuan.[2] He is normally referred to as Aged Ancestor Chen Tuan (陳搏老祖, Chen Tuan Lao Zu), and is also known as Chen Xiyi (陳希夷).

Born in 871 CE and died in 989, he lived from the end of the Five Dynasties and Ten Kingdoms period (907–960) and during the start of the Song dynasty (960–1279). He was possibly born in Luyi County, Henan Province. It is said he lived at Nine Chamber Cave (九室洞, Jiu Shi Dong) on Matchless Warrior Mountain (武當山, Wu Dang Shan), and later at Flower Mountain (華山, Hua Shan)—two famous sacred Taoist mountains.

---

[2] See *Life & Teachings of Two Immortals, Volume II, Chen Tuan* by Hua-Ching Ni (Seven Star Communications, 1993). Volume I of this series features Kou Hong (Ge Hong, author of the *Bao Pu Zi, Master Who Embraces Simplicity*).

In many ways, Chen Tuan is considered the father of what is now known as "Qigong" (氣功), a generic term used for describing all the various breathing and hygiene exercises developed within the Chinese teachings of Nourishing Life Arts. More correctly, Chen Tuan taught a series of exercises popularly known in his time as "Dao Yin" (道引), a Taoist term covering the methods of "Leading and Guiding Qi" through breathing, stretching, and self-massage techniques, and "Drawing-in and Spitting-out" (吐吶, Tu Na), a means of drawing in positive Yang Qi and expelling negative Yin Qi through the creation of sound, vibrations, and the release and expression of Qi.

His health and longevity regimes (presented in this work as the *Four Season Qigong* and *Twenty-Four Dao Yin Seated Exercises*) are in many ways similar to yoga practice. Not in the sense of being static postures, rather they are gestures of movements that accord with the breath so as to mobilize the Qi and target specific Qi meridians of the body.

Chen Tuan is also credited with a martial art style known as *Six Harmonies and Eight Methods* (六合八法, Liu He Ba Fa), another Qigong exercise called *Taiji Ruler* (太極尺, Tai Ji Shi), and a practice of supine meditation and Qigong, which gave him the moniker of the "Sleeping Immortal" (睡仙, Shui Xian).

Introduction

The exercises in this work are really quite simple and take little time to perform, just a few minutes each day, ten minutes or less two times daily. Despite the simplicity of their application, the benefits are numerous and the theories and correlations associated with them are extensive. Anyone sincerely engaging in these practices will not only find a trove of health benefits, but also acquire a more profound appreciation and understanding of Chen Tuan's truly brilliant work.

During my long tutelage with the great Taijiquan master T.T. Liang, he would frequently relate an old Chinese statement from Cheng Tang (成湯), the founder of the Shang dynasty (1776 BCE), who had the following verse engraved on his bathtubs: "Each day renew yourself, again renew, still renew, and always renew."

Anyone who consistently practices the exercise regimes in this work will gain the truth of Cheng Tang's verse, for that is what you are doing each and every day, *renewing*.

This work is a translation from an old Taoist text titled *The Book of Immortal Longevity of Ten Thousand Years* (萬壽仙書, *Wan Shou Xian Shu*), produced sometime around 1600 CE.[3] I also made use of the *Book of the Elixir of Good*

---

[3] See *Wan Shou Xian Shu: The Book of Immortal Longevity of Ten Thousand Years*, a reproduction of the Chinese work by Valley Spirit Arts, 2016.

Chen Tuan's Four Season Internal Kungfu

Fortune and Longevity (福壽丹書, *Fu Shou Dan Shu*), first published in 1621 CE, along with probably the most referenced book on this subject matter, the *Jade Tablet Decrees on Nature and Life,* first printed in 1650 CE. In addition, I borrowed greatly from *The Yellow Emperor's Internal Medicine Classic* (黃帝內經, *Huang Di Nei Jing*), written sometime around 320 BCE. I also used *The Secret Know-Hows of Refinement Skills* (練功秘訣, *Lian Gong Mi Jue*) by Sa Re (薩若), a reproduction of the 1600 CE edition, published in Taiwan in 1960. And, finally, I examined another work attributed to Chen Tuan dating back to the same era of 1600 CE, reproduced in Hong Kong in 1974 under the title *Seated Kung Illustrated and Explained* (坐功圖說, *Zuo Gong Tu Shuo*).

The Book of Immortal Longevity of Ten Thousand Years presents the Twenty-Four Seated Dao Yin Exercises, the Eight Brocades Dao Yin, the Five Animal Frolics, the Forty-Eight Medicinal Kung, and sections dealing with Taoist philosophy and practice. The *Book of the Elixir of Good Fortune and Longevity* contains the Four Season Qigong and Twenty-Four Seated Dao Yin Exercises, along with other information on herbs and Taoist theory of Nourishing Life Arts.

I reorganized the presentation of Chen Tuan's work into clear sections, as the original texts mostly just ran everything together or added relevant information to other sections. Many times I had to go to other sources to clarify certain statements. I have also added notes to explain some of the more cryptic and technical terms.

In comparison with the earliest transcriptions on the *Four Season Qigong,* later works appear to add material and exercises. I assume this was done so certain schools or teachers could implant their ideas and practices into the text and thereby gain the credentials of Chen Tuan, somewhat of a common practice in the formation of these types of Chinese works.

It's also the case that some additions were taken from one or more of the *Twenty-Four Dao Yin Seated Exercises* and placed with the *Four Season Qigong.* All such inclusions and variations can be confusing, and unnecessary, so I have kept the exercise explanations to adhere to the oldest, most traditional instructions.

Chen Tuan's Two Yearly Regimes

Chen Tuan's *Four Season Qigong* and *Twenty-Four Dao Yin Seated Exercises* are External Alchemy regimes designed for use during the four seasons and twenty-four lunar periods of the year. The "Four Season Seated Kung" (四季坐功, Si Ji Zuo Gong) relate to the positioning of the sun through the seasonal changes of the year, while the "Twenty-Four Qi Seated Kung Dao Yin Methods" (二十四氣坐功導引法, Er Shi Si Qi Zuo Gong Zhi Bing Fa) follow the twenty-four phases of the moon.

Each of the *Four Season Qigong* exercises are associated with one of the Four Celestial Animals of Taoist cosmology: *Green Dragon* with the springtime kung, *Red Bird* for summer, *White Tiger* for autumn, and Black Tortoise for winter. With the *Dao Yin Seated Exercises,* two exercises per month make twenty-four total in one year. They are performed on and during certain starting and ending dates (New Moon to Full Moon, and then Full Moon to New Moon) in accordance with the lunar calendar,[4] and are likewise advised to be practiced during the first four Chinese hours of the day for attaining the optimum benefit. In Chinese astrology, these times represent the hours of the Rat, Ox, Tiger, and Rabbit, and

---

[4] An online calendar showing the dates for performing the various exercises with the lunar cycle is available to Celestial Members of the Sanctuary of Tao (see sanctuaryoftao.org for more information).

because they mark the beginning periods of a new day they are classified as the "Ultimate Yang" hours of the day.[5]

There is really nothing too physically difficult with any of the exercises in this book, but they take focus and diligence. The regimes may not take much time to perform, but the periods indicated for doing them can be inconvenient. With that said, practicing them is most important. The designated time periods are beneficial, but not wholly critical, so whatever time you can practice them is fine.

Despite the simplicity of the exercises themselves, the theories, purposes, and medicinal benefits attached to them are complex and deep.

The exercise regimes are based on the two important Nourishing Life Arts of Dao Yin (導引) and Tu Na (吐呐). *Dao Yin* is primarily about the methods for circulating Qi in the body through specific body manipulations and movements. *Tu Na* covers the breathing methods used to accumulate and encourage the circulation of Qi. These practices begin as Waidan (stimulation of the external Qi), which then prepare the body for the Neidan stimulation of the internal Qi. Hence, the *Four Season Qigong* and the *Twenty-Four Dao Yin Seated Exercises* are a means of what Internal Alchemy teachings call Setting Up the Foundation (築基, Zhu Ji). Chen Tuan's methods here are primarily for health and longevity, yet they are the very precursors for the

---

[5] See Appendix, p. 311, for a list of the twelve animal signs and their associated hour of the day, month, and Earthly Branch.

Internal Alchemy practices and teachings leading to immortality.

Correlations with Chen Tuan's Two Yearly Regimes
Associating the *Four Season Qigong* and *Twenty-Four Dao Yin Seated Exercises* with sun and moon influences leads to a host of other important correlations with Chinese medicine and Taoist philosophy. Each of the Four Seasons relates to one of the Four Celestial Animals, and by extension to a specific organ of the body. The springtime, *Green Dragon,* exercises work to maintain the optimum health and function of the liver. The summer, *Red Bird,* exercises correlate to the heart; the autumn, *White Tiger,* exercises relate to the lungs; and the winter, *Black Tortoise,* exercises are for the kidneys.[6]

The liver, heart, lungs, and kidneys are the first four of the Five Viscera. The fifth, Triple Warmer (and spleen), is not ignored, however, as it is repaired, nourished, and strengthened consistently throughout the year within all the regimes of the *Twenty-Four Dao Yin Seated Exercises,* and from an assumed consistent practice of meditation. By affecting all Five Viscera, the Six Bowels (六腑, Liu Fu) are then regulated.

---

[6] The *Four Celestial Animals* were also given human names, probably to complete the correlation of them with the *Three Powers* (三才, San Cai) of *Heaven* (天, Tian, the Celestial), *Earth* (地, Di, the Terrestrial), and *Humanity* (人, Ren). See *Chart of the Five Forces Correlations* in the Appendix, p. 314.

The Four Celestial Animals are also representative of the Four Quadrants of the night sky. The *Twenty-Eight Constellations* are divided into four divisions with seven constellations (or mansions) indicated within them.

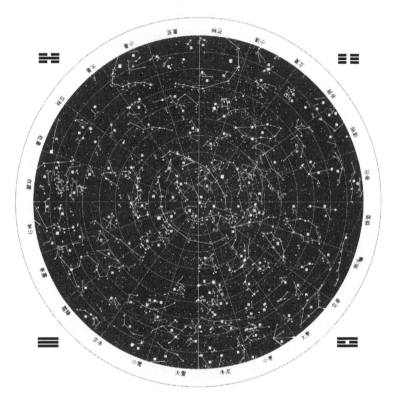

The *Four Quadrants* include *Green Dragon* (青龍, Qing Long) in the East (Fire ☲), *Black Tortoise* (玄武, Xuan Wu) in the North (Earth ☷), *White Tiger* (白虎, Bai Hu) in the West (Water ☵), and *Red Bird* (朱雀, Zhu Que) in the South (Heaven ☰).

Chen Tuan's Two Yearly Regimes

Even in the correlation with the Four Celestial Animals, the fifth celestial animal of the Yellow Dragon (黃龍, Huang Long) is implied (see *Late Summer* and *Long Summer* exercises), as it occupies the center of the Four Quadrants and represents Earth, spleen, and the Triple Warmer.

Book of Changes Associations

Like almost all Taoist works of this nature, Chen Tuan includes *Book of Changes* hexagram and trigram associations. It's not necessary to delve too deeply into this subject, as these associations can get complex. Suffice to say that each lunar month of the year is correlated with one of twelve hexagram images, called the *Twelve Lunar Sovereign Hexagrams*. These twelve images are not only associated with the months of the year, but also the Twelve Earthly Branches, and the twelve Chinese hours in each day.

The Twelve Lunar Sovereign Hexagrams

	#24	#19	#11	#34	#43	#1	#44	#33	#12	#20	#23	#2
	Fu	Lin	Tai	Da Zhuang	Guai	Qian	Gou	Dun	Pi	Guan	Bo	Kun
Earthly Branch	子	丑	寅	卯	辰	巳	午	未	申	酉	戌	亥
	Zi	Chou	Yin	Mao	Chen	Si	Wu	Wei	Shen	You	Xu	Hai
Twelve Animals	Rat	Ox	Tiger	Rabbit	Dragon	Snake	Horse	Goat	Monkey	Rooster	Dog	Pig
Month	11	12	1	2	3	4	5	6	7	8	9	10
Hour	23-1	1-3	3-5	5-7	7-9	9-11	11-13	13-15	15-17	17-19	19-21	21-23

These twelve hexagrams not only relate to the lunar months of the year, but they are used in Internal Alchemy to indicate the process of Qi movement (mobilization of the Qi) within the body throughout the twelve periods of the day, called *Firing Times* in some texts.

If looking up the images for the Spring Season Internal Kungfu and Dao Yin exercises, for example, you can see that they are images #11, #34, and #43, the first three months of the year. Their Earthly Branch associations are Yin (Tiger), Mao (Rabbit), and Chen (Dragon).

At first, understanding these associations is not crucial to the practice or for benefiting from the *Qigong* and *Dao Yin* exercises. After gaining some insight into the *Book of Changes*, however, and studying associations with it, as well as the other correlations with Chen Tuan's works, you'll gain a much deeper and spiritual understanding of the practices.[7]

---

[7] See the Appendix and the *Book of Sun and Moon (I Ching)*, volumes I and II (Valley Spirit Arts, 2014) for more information on the *Book of Changes* and the numerous correlations with it.

The Six Zi and Classifications of Qi Influences

Taoist texts refer to six celestial vibrational energies in the universe and the human body. Termed as *Ultimate Yang, Ultimate Yin, Young Yang, Young Yin, Bright Yang,* and *Faint Yin,* these six terms (Six Zi) are associated with everything from classifications of Qi, to the meridian systems of Chinese medicine and Internal Alchemy, to astrological calculations, *Book of Changes* imagery (within trigrams and hexagrams, casting of images, and so on), to elemental activities, and the influences of the climate and excessive energy within the body.

In Chen Tuan's text describing the *Twenty-Four Dao Yin Seated Exercises,* these six terms have different meanings of expression. In the first verse of each exercise, for example, he uses them as a type of Qi energy classification. Whereas in the second verse, he is using them to reference one of the Twelve Primary Qi Meridians (i.e., *Bright Yang Hand Meridian).* The first verse, then, is referencing them in their Yin and Yang atmospheric, or worldly, energetic ideal and philosophical sense, while the second verse is referring to the physiological expression the Yin and Yang vibrational energies take in the body via meridians.

Starting the first verse of each of the *Twenty-Four Dao Yin Seated Exercises* with the three simple words of

"Mobilize and control" implies a great deal of meaning and purpose for each of the exercises.

Mobilize (運, Yun) means "to move and revolve the Qi/breath." *Control* (主, Zhu) means "to master or rule over," or simply the idea of "directing the Qi." Together, this compound of *Yun Zhu* (運主) is expressing the idea that the exercises "control and regulate the circulation of Qi."

The next part in the verse addresses the type of Qi the exercise is seeking to mobilize and control. The distinctions of *New Qi, Two Qi, Three Qi, Four Qi,* or *Five Qi,* express the idea of Qi as "the influences of nature's forces," and Chen Tuan is referencing these classifications of Qi within his instructions to point out the stages and effects of the serious cultivation of these exercises.

Within the texts of the *Four Season Qigong* and *Twenty-Four Dao Yin Seated Exercises,* Chen Tuan does not mention the classification of "One Qi,"[8] as this designation is reserved for the Internal Alchemy practice of the Lesser Heavenly Circuit, wherein the goal is to achieve this "One Breath" skill. For reasons of clarification, it is included here.

---

8   See *Refining the Elixir: The Internal Alchemy Teachings of Taoist Immortal Zhang Sanfeng* (Valley Spirit Arts, 2016) for a deeper analysis of "One Qi," as the subject is quite extensive.

The Six Zi and Classifications of Qi Influences

One Qi (一氣, Yi Qi, the "One Breath" or "Action"). In Taoism, the "One Qi" is an expression of Tao, as each breath is the Tao.⁹ In other Taoist interpretations, One Qi is interpreted to mean the Illimitable (無極, Wu Ji), represented by an empty circle.

In expressing the importance of the "One Breath," the Yellow Emperor, Huang Di, once said, "With each inhalation, the Ten Heavenly Stems are taken in, and with each exhalation, the Twelve Earthly Branches are released."¹⁰

---

9   Many Taoists books, and even some Buddhist ones, include the term *Chen Tuan's Great Reason* (陳搏大因, Chen Tuan Da Yin), which basically means the attainment of Tao through the methods taught by Chen Tuan. The *Great Reason* method refers to the sublimation of True Mercury, True Lead, Original Spirit, Mind-Intention, and Original Essence, which are all components of the Elixir of Immortality. All five components are contained within each breath we take, but only through dedicated cultivation are we able to perceive this *Great Reason*.

10 The *Ten Heavenly Stems* (十天干, Shi Tian Gan) are formed on the combination of the Five Elements in both their Yin and Yang aspects (meaning, there are five Yang types of Fire, Wood, Earth, Metal, and Water, and five Yin ones). The *Twelve Earthly Branches* (十二地支, Shi Er Di Zhi) are representative of the twelve months of a year. When used together, such as in Huang Di's quote, they are also referring to the Sixty-Year Cycle of the Chinese calendar—which is calculated by multiplying the Five Elements (or Stems) by the Twelve Earthly Branches in each year, which amounts to sixty. Huang Di's quote, then, is another way of giving importance to this idea of "One Breath," because he's implying that all Sixty Cycles are completed within it. See Appendix for more information on these subjects.

New Qi (初氣) is a term associated with the advent of spring, experienced in nature as well as within the human body. In spring, the Qi of the body begins a regeneration process as the more stagnant period of winter passes. Many old Taoist texts express this idea in the statement, "Breathe in the spring and exhale the winter" (呼春吸冬, Hu Chun Xi Dong). New Qi is also likened to the idea of breathing in the Before Heaven Qi and exhaling the After Heaven Qi,[11] or *inhaling the Ten Heavenly Stems and exhaling the Twelve Earthly Branches*. Basically, it is the idea of breathing in New Yang Qi and exhaling the Old (Faint) Yin Qi of the body.

Two Qi (二氣) comes from the metaphor of the "two Qi of the dragon and tiger elixir" (二氣龍虎丹), or even more simply *Yin* and *Yang*. The elixir being the components of Jing (精, Essence, Tiger, and Yin), and Qi (氣, Vital Energy, Dragon, and Yang). The body is divided into these two areas of influence by Yin and Yang (or Dragon and Tiger), or as in the Taiji Symbol, divisions of Yin (black) and Yang (white). The left side is Yang, the right Yin. The back of the body is Yang, the front Yin. The

---

[11] *Before Heaven Qi* (先天氣, Xian Tian Qi) refers to prenatal conditions and Innate Breathing. *After Heaven Qi* (後天氣, Hou Tian Qi) refers to postnatal conditions and Acquired Breathing. The basic premise is that *Before Heaven Breath* is how we breathed in our mother's womb, and *After Heaven Breath* is how we breathe after the umbilical cord is severed.

The Six Zi and Classifications of Qi Influences

and the interior Yin. Just as the External Elixir (Waidan) is a Yang process, and Internal Elixir (Neidan) is a Yin process.

Yin and Yang in the Taiji Symbol

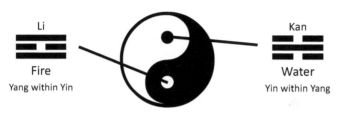

As stated in *The Yellow Emperor's Internal Medicine Classic*, "The purpose of the external Yang is to support the internal Yin." This statement is full of meaning, but for the subject of this book, it means using the resources of Waidan to bring about the effects of Neidan, or as Taoist Internal Alchemy books state, to "Use the After Heaven to bring about the Before Heaven."

On just a purely physiological interpretation, *dragon* and *tiger* can be referring to the liver and lungs, as it is crucial in the spring months to repair, nourish, and strengthen these two organs.

Three Qi has variant meanings. In one sense it's defined through three philosophical terms that relate to the Three Treasures (三寶, San Bao):
1. "Mysteriousness (玄, Xuan) of Life" relates to Shen.
2. "Greatness (元, Yuan) of Life" relates to Qi.
3. "Origin (始, Shi) of Life" relates to Jing.

In other words, the *Shen* is defined as the energy of the Mysterious Nature of Life, the *Qi* is defined as the energy that gives Greatness to Life, and *Jing* is defined as the energy that is the very Source of Life.

Visually, the Three Qi aspects are represented in the Taiji Symbol. Along with the major Yin and Yang divisions of the symbol representing two Qi, the inclusion of the small Yin and Yang circles within their opposite represents the third Qi. Or as Lao Zi points out, "The One begets the Two, and the Two beget Three."

In physiological terms, the Three Qi is referring to the three divisions of the Triple Warmer, an ethereal organ that provides body warmth and Qi to the head, trunk, and lower regions of the body, and also affects the endocrine and exocrine systems and functions of the body. The Triple Warmer controls the passageways of heat and fluids in the body, and so controls the function and production of the saliva (which is stimulated within each of the *Twenty-Four Dao Yin Seated Exercises)* to support the activities of the Earth element.

Four Qi (四氣, Si Qi) is a reference to the Qi of the liver, heart, lungs, and kidneys—the four essentials of life. *The Yellow Emperor's Internal Medicine Classic* states, "Planting and production accord with the spring [Wood Element] months; growing and cultivating accord with the summer [Fire] months; gathering and harvesting accord with the

The Six Zi and Classifications of Qi Influences

autumn [Metal] months; and storage of the crops accord with the winter [Water] months."

Physiologically, the Qi of the liver is expressed in the activities associated with the element of Wood; the Qi of the heart, with the activities of Fire; the Qi of the lungs, with the activities of Metal; and the Qi of the kidneys, with the activities of Water.

The Four Qi can also be interpreted on a visual basis as the Four Pillar Images of the *Book of Changes:*

☰ (乾, Qian) meaning Heaven (or Sky).

☷ (坤, Kun) meaning Earth (or Soil).

☲ (離, Li) meaning Fire (or Sun).

☵ (坎, Kan) meaning Water (or Moon).

These four images play heavily in the processes of Internal Alchemy.

Five Qi (五氣, Wu Qi) is a reference to the energies of Essence (精, Jing), Spirit (神, Shen), Heavenly Spirit (魂, Hun), Earthly Spirit (魄, Po), and Mind-Intent (意, Yi). In a purely physiological interpretation, the Five Qi are the liver, heart, spleen, lungs, and kidneys, but in this case the meaning extends to the optimum health and functions of the Five Viscera, wherein the Qi has been absorbed into and permeates each organ.

The Five Qi are also referred to in Internal Alchemy practice as the Five Forces (五力, Wu Li). The Five Forces are the five elemental activities of Earth, Metal, Water, Wood, and Fire along with their Yin and Yang aspects, as seen in the Ten Heavenly Stems of Chinese astrology. Here is a brief summary of the stems and their meanings on nature and Internal Alchemy and their associated season of the year:

Ten Heavenly Yin and Yang Stems

Jia (甲, 1st stem) is **Yang Wood** and is likened to forests and trees in nature. **Yi** (乙, 2nd stem) is **Yin Wood,** likened to small plants and flowers. Jia with *Zi* (子, first of the Twelve Earthly Branches) means *Beginning of Spring.* Yi with *Hai* (亥, last of the Twelve Earthly Branches) means *End of Spring.*

In Internal Alchemy, Yang and Yin Wood represent the correlations associated with True Mercury (Heavenly Spirit, Hun), the celestial animal *Green Dragon,* Inner Nature, the liver, the color green, and the easterly direction.

Bing (丙, 3rd stem) is **Yang Fire** and is likened to the sun. **Ding** (丁, 4th stem) is **Yin Fire** and likened to fires and flames. Bing Zi means *Beginning of Summer.* Ding Hai is *End of Summer.*

Yang and Yin Fire represent the correlations associated with the Cinnabar (Before Heaven Qi), the celestial animal *Red Bird,* Original Spirit, the heart, the color red, and the southerly direction.

Wu (戊, 5th stem) is **Yang Earth** and is likened to boulders and rocks. **Ji** (己, 6th stem) is **Yin Earth** and is likened to soil and farmed fields. Wu is associated with *Late Summer*; Ji with *Long Summer*. Earth is the center of the Five Activities and therefore not assigned a season, rather as the fluctuation that occurs in a year with a summer season that comes late after spring, or a summer that extends into the autumn season. Therefore, these can either become a *Late Summer* of Ding Zi or a *Long Summer* of Geng Zi.

Yang and Yin Earth represent the correlations associated with the Elixir, the Celestial Cauldron (where the Four Celestial Animals converge), Mind-Intention, the spleen, the color yellow, and the central position.

Geng (庚, 7th stem) is **Yang Metal** and is likened to steel and swords. **Xin** (辛, 8th stem) is **Yin Metal,** likened to gold and silver. Yang and Yin Metal represent the correlations associated with True Lead, the celestial animal *White Tiger,* emotions (Earthly Spirit, Po), the lungs, the color white, and the westerly direction. Geng Zi means *Beginning of Autumn.* Xin Hai means *End of Autumn.*

Ren (壬, 9th stem) is **Yang Water,** likened to rivers and oceans. **Gui** (癸, 10th stem) is **Yin Water,** likened to rain and dew. Ren Zi means *Beginning of Winter.* Gui Hai means *End of Winter.*

Yang and Yin Water represent the correlations associated with Original Essence (Before Heaven Jing), the celestial animal *Black Tortoise,* the kidneys, the color black, and the northerly direction.

When the Five Forces are refined and united, *Returning Spirit to the Void* can occur.

Lastly, for the two main types of Qi, Chen Tuan uses the terms **Bright Yang Qi** (陽明氣, Yang Ming Qi) and **Faint Yin Qi** (厥陰氣, Jue Yin Qi). *Bright Yang Qi* can be thought of like the sun and *Faint Yin Qi* like the moon, a contrast between light and dark, and to the double fish images (white and dark divisions) in the Taiji Symbol. Within us the Qi moves naturally in a cycle of Yang and Yin, moving from *Bright Yang* to *Faint Yin* within each twenty-four hour period. These two terms signify the change that takes place when either the Yang Qi or Yin Qi reaches its peak and reverts to the other. Like how the sun's rising and setting each day gives way to the moon's rising and setting each night.

The associations continue with the correlations of the *Six Qi* (六氣, the six conditions of climate—*cold, wind, heat, moisture, fire,* and *drought*), the *Seven Qi* (七氣, Qi Qi, Seven Earthly Spirits or Emotions), the *Eight Qi* (八氣, Ba Qi, Eight Diagrams, ☰ ☱ ☲ ☳ ☴ ☵ ☶ ☷), and *Nine Qi* (九氣, Nine Palaces and Nine Restorations).[12]

In brief, Chen Tuan's use of these terms in the text is showing that in the spring season, the energy of New Qi is first cultivated, and then the energies of the Two Qi (Yin/

---

12 See *Refining the Elixir* and *Book of Sun and Moon (I Ching),* volumes I and II (Valley Spirit Arts, 2014) for information on *Seven Qi, Eight Qi,* and *Nine Qi.*

The Six Zi and Classifications of Qi Influences

Tiger and Yang/Dragon) take over. This period is called *Sprouting Qi*.

In the summer season, the Qi of the Three Treasures (Jing, Qi, and Shen) are being cultivated—called *Growing Qi*.

In autumn, the Qi of the Four Images of Heaven (☰), Earth (☷), Water (☵), and Fire (☲) are cultivated—called *Harvesting Qi*.

In winter, the Qi of the Five Activities (Earth, Metal, Water, Wood, and Fire) are cultivated. This phase is termed as *Storing Qi*.

At this point, the Qi of the *Ultimate Yang* is present, but it will revert to *Faint Yin* if the Qi is not mobilized for the undertaking of Internal Alchemy.

The following summary outlines the progression of Qi classifications as they appear within the yearly practices of the *Four Season Qigong* and *Twenty-Four Dao Yin Seated Exercises*.[13]

New Qi (初氣, Chu Qi): occurs in the first full moon of the year, *Green Dragon Kung* and Dao Yin exercises 1 and 2.

Two Qi (二氣, Er Qi): starts in the second moon of *Green Dragon Kung*, but concludes after the first half moon

---

13   Each season (and Kung) is three lunar months and coincides with six Dao Yin exercises, so the *Green Dragon Kung* includes Dao Yin exercises 1 thru 6. *Red Bird Kung* covers 7 thru 12. *White Tiger,* 13 thru 18. *Black Tortoise,* 19 thru 24.

of *Red Bird Kung*. Appears five times in Dao Yin exercises 3 thru 7.

Three Qi (三氣, San Qi): begins in the last half of the first summer moon, *Red Bird Kung*, and concludes in the first half of the third summer moon. Appears four times in Dao Yin exercises 8 thru 11.

Four Qi (四氣, Si Qi): starts in the final half moon of *Red Bird Kung* and concludes in the first half of autumn's second moon, *White Tiger Kung*. Appears four times in Dao Yin exercises 12 thru 15.

Five Qi (五氣, Wu Qi): starts in the last half of the second moon of *White Tiger Kung* and ends after the first half moon of *Black Tortoise Kung*. Appears four times in Dao Yin exercises 16 thru 19.

Ultimate Yang Qi (太陽氣, Tai Yang Qi): from the second half of the first winter moon, *Black Tortoise Kung*, the Qi of *Ultimate Yang* is sought and concludes in the first half of the third winter moon. Appears four times in Dao Yin exercises 20 thru 23.

Faint Yin Qi (厥陰氣, Jue Yin Qi): in the final half of the third winter month, the Qi of *Faint Yin* returns, appearing just once with Dao Yin exercise 24.

Come the New Year, the *New Qi* arrives and the cycle starts anew.

The Six Zi and Classifications of Qi Influences

The point of Internal Alchemy rests in the experience of remaining in this state of *Ultimate Yang Qi,* for which the exercises in this work are directed.

As stated earlier, working through Chen Tuan's regimes and experiencing the varying stages of Qi development is the process of Setting Up the Foundation of Internal Alchemy. Whether a person can accomplish this in just a one-year cycle, or it means taking many years of repeated effort, there's no guarantee. Once the effects of *Ultimate Yang Qi* are experienced, this is the point in which to move on to Internal Alchemy practices to accomplish what Chen Tuan calls the *Great Reason* (大因, Da Yin)—his way of saying "Entering the Tao."

Six Zi and The Twelve Primary Qi Meridians

The second verse for each of the *Twenty-Four Dao Yin Seated Exercises* lists the name of the Qi meridian being stimulated in the exercise. There are fourteen major Qi meridians of the body, of which the Twelve Primary Yin and Yang Meridians directly relate to the exercises in this work. Each of these twelve meridians, in both hand and foot types, appear twice in the exercises.[14]

The six hand meridians are assigned to the first six months of the year and the six foot meridians are used in the last six months, correlating to the Yin and Yang divisions of hands being Yang and the feet being Yin.

In chapter 11 of *The Yellow Emperor's Internal Medicine Classic,* under the section "Spiritual Pivot" (靈樞, Ling Shu), appears the following statement on meridians:

There are six celestial vibration patterns [Six Zi],
and from these the Yin and Yang meridian system
within the human body is established. These [twelve
meridians] directly correlate with the twelve months
of the year, the twelve Earthly Branches, the twelve

---

[14] *Ultimate Yang Hand* is referenced three times, but in the first case it is in combination with the *Young Yang Hand* (Triple Warmer) Meridian (see Dao Yin Exercise 1). *Young Yang Hand* is mentioned by itself only once in Exercise 2.

divisions of the sky, the twelve rivers, and the twelve time periods of the day. The twelve meridians, therefore, represent the fixed way in which the organ systems of the human body receive their functionality, and so resonate with the Heavenly Tao.

These "six celestial vibration patterns" equate to the Six Zi, and are comprised of three Yang meridians and three Yin meridians.

The Yang Meridians
Ultimate Yang
 (太陽, Tai Yang)
Young Yang
 (少陽, Shao Yang)
Bright Yang
 (陽明, Yang Ming)

The Yin Meridians
Ultimate Yin
 (太陰, Tai Yin)
Young Yin
 (少陰, Shao Yin)
Faint Yin
 (厥陰, Jue Yin)

From these six meridians come the further classifications of Hand (手, Shou) and Foot (足, Zu) types, depending on where each meridian runs in the body. In total, they form the Twelve Primary External Yin and Yang Meridians (six hand meridians and six foot meridians).

The Dumai (毒脈) and Renmai (任脈) meridians are not mentioned in the exercises as they come into play within the External Elixir practices of stimulating the Lesser Heavenly Circuit[15] through meditation practice. Actually,

---

15 *Lesser Heavenly Circuit* (小天周, Xiao Tian Zhou) is sometimes called the "Microcosmic Orbit."

Six Zi and the Twelve Primary Qi Meridians

the Dumai and Renmai are the most important, as they control all the Yin and Yang meridians of the body.[16]

Although only the Twelve Primary Meridians are referenced within the exercise instructions, the stimulation of these meridians will naturally produce effects within the Dumai and Renmai meridians, and a practitioner can expect to periodically sense heat rising up the spine and down the front of the body. This sensation is a result of the External Elixir (or Qi) mobilizing in the body, but should not be confused with the more fluid-like sensations of the Internal Elixir.

The drawings in this section on the meridians and the classical illustrations shown in the *Four Season Qigong* and *Twenty-Four Dao Yin Seated Exercises* have some slight differences, such as the number of designated Qi points indicated with certain meridians. Also keep in mind that the Twelve Primary Meridians are bilateral, which means they have symmetrical pathways on each side of the body in relation to the mid-line of the body. The Qi points for the various meridians are in the same locations on both sides of the body, and some drawings will indicate the mirror-image Qi points for reference purposes. Also, one drawing of a meridian may show the path on the left arm, for example, while the classical version may show it on the right side.

---

[16] The meridian references here are to Waidan, not Internal Elixir. In both systems the names and locations for the Qi meridians are the same, but in function completely different. See *Refining the Elixir* for more information.

This makes no difference in terms of the actual paths of the meridians and the Qi points along them.

Ultimate Yang Meridians

1. Ultimate Yang Hand (手太陽, Shou Tai Yang) is connected with the vessels and cavities supporting the small intestine (小腸, xiao chang), so is called the Small Intestine Meridian, and is governed by the elemental activity of Fire. It enjoins with the Heart Meridian.

Official name: Minister of Cleansing.

Traditional name: Ultimate Yang Hand Small Intestine Meridian.

Function: the small intestine receives and processes food by separating out nutrients and waste, with the nutrients becoming bodily fluids and the waste becoming urine. This meridian is responsible for digestion, water absorption, nutrient absorption, and bowel functions.

Peak Hour of Function: Goat (1:00 to 3:00 p.m.)

Meridian Pathway: the Qi of this meridian flows up the back of the arm and into the head. It begins in the Qi point of *Young Marsh* (少澤, Shao Ze, SI-1) and ends in the *Listening Palace* (聽宮, Ting Gong, SI-19).

The Ultimate Yang Hand Meridian begins at the lateral tip of the little finger and then runs along the side of the hand over the wrist and along the rear side of the forearm until arriving and curving over the back of the shoulder. Then, from the uppermost part of the back at the base of the neck, it moves across the neck and up into the cheek until it changes direction under the eye to complete the path in front of the ear.

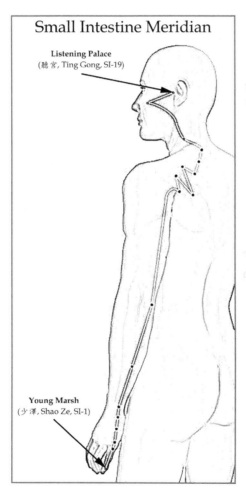

2. Ultimate Yang Foot (足太陽, Zu Tai Yang) is connected with the vessels and cavities supporting the urinary bladder, and so is called the Bladder Meridian. It is governed by the elemental activity of Water and enjoins with the Kidney Meridian.

Official name: Guardian of Peace.

Traditional name: Ultimate Yang Foot Urinary Bladder Meridian.

Function: the Bladder Meridian is intrinsically related to the functions and balance of the autonomous nervous system, which regulates all the body's basic vital functions. The urinary bladder as an organ is responsible for the storage and removal of urine.

Peak Hour of Function: Monkey (3:00 to 5:00 p.m.)

Meridian Pathway: the Qi of this meridian flows downward from the head through the back of the body and ends in the foot. It is the longest and most complex of all the meridians, beginning in the Qi point of *Bright Eye* (睛明, Jing Ming, UB-1) and ending in *Foremost Yin* (至陰, Zhi Yin, UB-67).

This meridian starts at the inner canthus of the eye and travels over the forehead to the back of the head. At the occiput it forms two branches that travel down the back to the lumbar region. From there it descends along the posterior aspect of the thigh to the back of the knee joint, then descends through the calf muscle and further to the outer side of the ankle and foot, ending at the outside tip of the little toe.

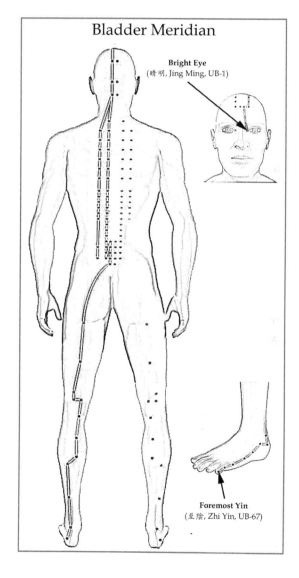

Ultimate Yin Meridians

3. Ultimate Yin Hand (手太陰, Shou Tai Yin) is connected with the vessels and cavities supporting the lungs. Called the Lung Meridian, it is governed by the elemental activity of Metal.

Official name: Minister of Body and Mind.

Traditional name: Ultimate Yin Hand Lung Meridian.

Function: Controls breath and vitality. It connects with the Large Intestine Meridian and assists with the circulation of blood.

Peak Hour of Function: Tiger (3:00 to 5:00 a.m.)

Meridian Pathway: The Qi in this meridian first flows upward from the solar plexus and then down the arm from the shoulder. The meridian begins in the shoulder in the Qi point of *Central Mansion* (中府, Zhong Fu, Lu-1) and ends on the thumb in the Qi point *Young Consulter* (少商, Shao Shang, Lu-11).

This meridian begins deep in the solar plexus region of the Middle Triple Warmer and descends to meet the Large Intestine Meridian. Moving up past the stomach, it crosses the diaphragm, divides, and enters the lungs. It then rejoins, passes up the middle of the windpipe to the throat and divides again, surfacing in the hollow region near the front of the shoulder (Lu-1). From here it passes over the shoulder and down the front of the arm along the outer border of the biceps muscle. It continues down the forearm to the wrist just above the base of the thumb. The channel crosses the height of the thumb muscle to finish at the corner of the thumbnail.

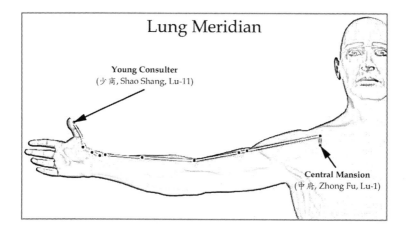

4. Ultimate Yin Foot (足太陰, Zu Tai Yin) is connected with the vessels and cavities supporting the spleen, so is called the Spleen Meridian. It is governed by the elemental activity of Earth.

Official name: Minister of Open Mindedness.
Traditional name: Ultimate Yin Foot Spleen Meridian.

Function: This meridian controls the salivary glands and the production of blood in the flesh of the body. It is enjoined with the Stomach Meridian.

Peak Hour of Function: Snake (9:00 to 11:00 a.m.)

Meridian Pathway: The Qi in this meridian flows upward from the foot to the head. It begins in the Qi point of *Hidden White* (隱白, Yin Bai, Sp-1) and ends in *Great Control* (大包, Da Bao, Sp-21).

The Ultimate Yin Foot Meridian starts at the tip of the big toe. From there it runs along the medial aspect of the foot at the junction of the inner ankle bone. It then continues upward along the inner leg, up across the side of the groin, the stomach, and through the diaphragm, where it then joins with the Stomach Meridian and Heart Meridian.

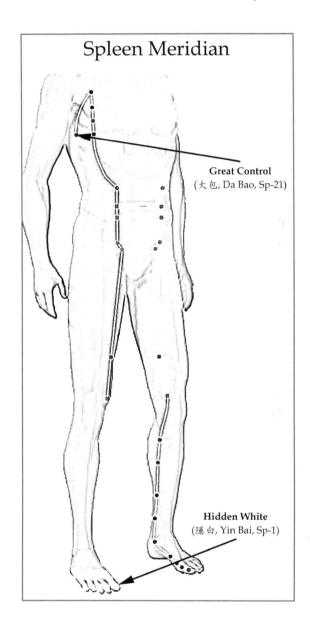

Young Yang Meridians

5. Young Yang Hand (手少陽, Shou Shao Yang) is connected with the vessels and cavities supporting the Triple Warmer, and so is called the Triple Warmer Meridian. It is governed by the elemental activity of Fire, and is enjoined with the Pericardium Meridian.

Official name: Minister of Transformation.

Traditional name: Young Yang Hand Triple Warmer Meridian.

Function: the Triple Warmer Meridian controls the movement and conversion of various solids and fluids throughout the circulatory and endocrine systems of the body, as well as for the production and circulation of nourishing and protective Qi. As a functional energy system of the body, it regulates the activities of all the other organs. The Triple Warmer is composed of three sections—thorax, abdomen, and pelvis—called Burners or Heaters. The Upper Burner controls intake, the Middle Burner controls conversion, and the Lower Burner controls elimination.

Peak Hour of Function: Pig (9:00 to 11:00 p.m.)

Meridian Pathway: the Qi of this meridian flows upwards through the back of the arm and into the head. It begins in the Qi point of *Pass Rinse* (關沖, Guan Chong, SJ-1) and ends in the *Silk Bamboo Opening* (絲竹空, Si Zhu Kong, SJ-23).

Six Zi and the Twelve Primary Qi Meridians

The Triple Warmer Meridian originates in the tip of the ring finger, by the outside corner of the nail, passes between the knuckles of the fourth and fifth fingers, and on to the wrist. From there it ascends between the two bones of the forearm (radius and ulna), through the tip of the elbow, and up the back of the arm to the shoulder. It moves forward into the chest to connect with the pericardium, the Upper Burner, the abdomen, and the Middle and Lower burners. Re-emerging from the chest at the collarbone, the meridian ascends the side of the neck and travels around the back of the ear.

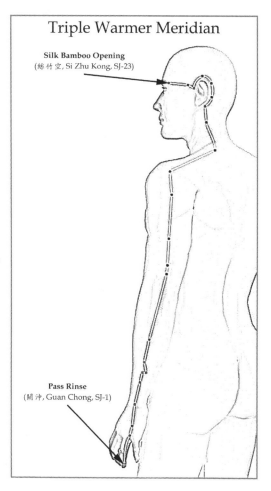

Triple Warmer Meridian

Silk Bamboo Opening
(絲竹空, Si Zhu Kong, SJ-23)

Pass Rinse
(關沖, Guan Chong, SJ-1)

6. *Young Yang Foot* (足少陽, Zu Shao Yang) is connected with the vessels and cavities supporting the gallbladder, so is called the Gallbladder Meridian. It is governed by the elemental activity of Wood and is enjoined with the Liver Meridian.

Official name: Guardian of Courage.

Traditional name: Young Yang Foot Gallbladder Meridian.

Function: The energy flow of this meridian's Qi controls our decision making process and the ability to make good and clear judgments. Among many other mental functions this meridian when functioning well gives us courage and initiative.

Peak Hour of Function: Rat (11:00 p.m. to 1:00 a.m.)

Meridian Pathway: the meridian begins in the Qi point of *Moonlight Crevice* (瞳子髎, Tong Zi Liao, GB-1) and ends with *Yin Foot Cavity* (足竅陰, Zu Qiao Yin, GB-44). The Qi flow of this meridian circles across the side of the head then descends the body to end in the foot.

This meridian begins just outside the outer corner of the eye, turns down towards the ear and then up into the forehead just along the hair line. From here it descends behind the ear.

It then moves back to the forehead above the center of the eye and moving down the head to the bottom of the skull. It continues down the neck into the shoulder, and then descends to the side of the body along the ribs, and into the waist and pelvis. It continues down the outside of the leg to the ankle, ending on the outside of the fourth toe.

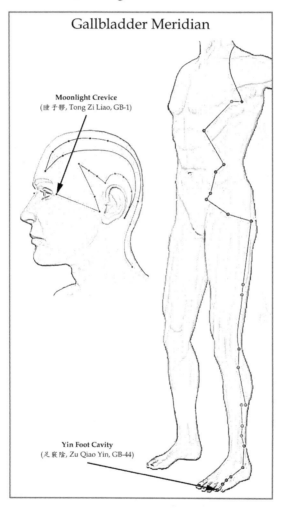

Young Yin Meridians

7. Young Yin Hand (手少陰, Shou Shao Yin) is connected with the vessels and cavities supporting the heart, so is called the Heart Meridian. It is governed by the elemental activity of Fire and reveals itself through brightness in the eyes.

Official name: Minister of Illumination.
Traditional name: Young Yin Hand Heart Meridian.

Function: This meridian controls the circulation of blood and its vessels (arteries, veins, and capillaries). It's enjoined with the Small Intestine Meridian.

Peak Hour of Function: Horse (11:00 a.m. to 1:00 p.m.)

Meridian Pathway: the Qi of this meridian flows upwards through the chest and then downwards along the inner arm. It begins in the Qi point of *Ultimate Well* (極泉, Ji Quan, H-1) and ends in *Little Rinse* (少沖, Shao Chong, H-9).

The Young Yin Hand Meridian originates from the heart, emerges and spreads over the heart system, passes through the diaphragm to connect with the Small Intestine. The exterior (surface) part runs over the lung, then turns downward along the arm. It ends in the inner tip of the little finger.

Six Zi and the Twelve Primary Qi Meridians

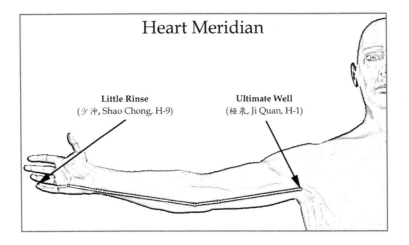

8. Young Yin Foot (足少陰, Zu Shao Yin) is connected with the vessels and cavities supporting the kidneys, so is called the Kidney Meridian. It is governed by the elemental activity of Water. When this meridian is functioning properly it reveals itself through clarity of mind and active energy of the body.

Official name: Minister of Courage.
Traditional name: Young Yin Foot Kidney Meridian.

Function: This meridian controls the growth and development of bones and nourishes the marrow, which is the body's source of red and white blood cells. It enjoins with the Bladder Meridian.

Peak Hour of Function: Rooster (5:00 to 7:00 p.m.)

Meridian Pathway: The Qi of this meridian flows upward from the bottom of the foot and into the head. It begins in the Qi point of *Bubbling Well* (湧泉, Yong Quan, K-1) and ends in *Shu Mansion* (俞府, Shu Fu, K-27).

The Young Yin Foot Meridian begins at the bottom of the foot, moves up the inner side of the ankle and the inner side of the leg. It passes through the groin area and up the torso and chest, ending near the clavicle.

Six Zi and the Twelve Primary Qi Meridians

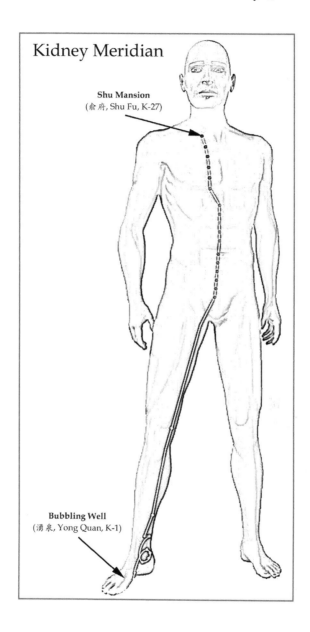

Bright Yang Meridians

9. Bright Yang Hand (手陽明, Shou Yang Ming) is connected with the vessels and cavities supporting the large intestine, so is called the Large Intestine Meridian. It is governed by the elemental activity of Metal.

Official name: Minister of Transportation.

Traditional name: Bright Yang Hand Large Intestine Meridian.

Function: This meridian controls the transformation of digestive wastes from liquid to solid state and transports the solids outward for excretion through the rectum. It plays a major role in the balance and purity of bodily fluids and assists the lungs in controlling the skin's pores and perspiration. It is enjoined with the Lung Meridian.

Peak Hour of Function: Rabbit (5:00 to 7:00 a.m.)

Meridian Pathway: the Qi of this meridian flows upwards from the hand, through the shoulder, and into the face. The meridian begins in the Qi point of *Consulting Yang* (商陽, Shang Yang, LI-1) and ends in *Welcoming Fragrance* (迎香, Ying Xiang, LI-20).

The Bright Yang Hand Meridian begins on the outside corner of the index fingernail. It then runs along the edge of the finger, between the two tendons of the thumb at the wrist joint and along the outer edge of the arm to the elbow. It continues to the outside of the shoulder muscle, then crosses the shoulder blade and travels upward over the muscle at the side of the neck to the cheek, passing through the lower gums, then over the top lip and ends beside the outer nostril.

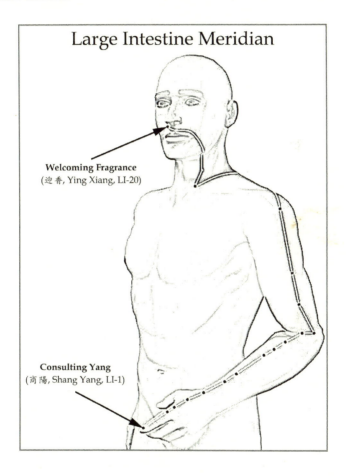

10. Bright Yang Foot (足陽明, Zu Yang Ming) is connected with the vessels and cavities supporting the stomach, so is called the Stomach Meridian, and is governed by the elemental activity of Earth.

Official name: Minister of Nourishment.
Traditional name: Bright Yang Foot Stomach Meridian.

Function: This meridian controls the assimilation of Qi absorbed and digested from food in conjunction with the Spleen Meridian.
Peak Hour of Function: Dragon (7:00 to 9:00 a.m.)

Meridian Pathway: the Qi of this meridian flows downward from the side of the head, through the torso and into the leg and foot.

The meridian begins in the Qi point of *Weeping Receiver* (承泣, Cheng Qi, St-1) and ends in *History Valley* (歷兌, Li Dui, St-45).

The Bright Yang Foot Meridian starts between the lower eyelid and the eye socket, and runs down the face and looping up to the forehead. From alongside the head it backtracks down and across to the shoulder, down the ribs along the stomach, and then down the leg along the anterior aspect of the thigh and reaching the knee. From there it continues down along the lateral aspect of the tibia to the top of the foot and reaches the lateral side of the tip of the second toe.

Six Zi and the Twelve Primary Qi Meridians

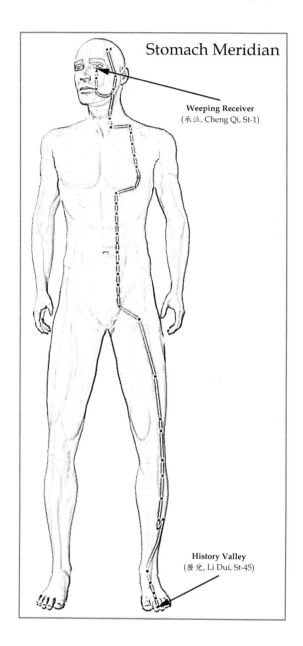

Faint Yin Meridians

11. Faint Yin Hand (手厥陰, Shou Jue[17] Yin) is connected with the vessels and cavities supporting the pericardium, so is called the Pericardium Meridian. It's governed by the elemental activities of Fire, and is enjoined with the Triple Warmer Meridian, also called the Triple Energizer or Burner Meridian.

Official name: Guardian of the Heart.

Traditional name: Faint Yin Hand Pericardium Meridian.

Function: the pericardium provides the heart with physical protection. Its energy also protects the heart from damage and disruption by excessive emotional energies generated by the other organs, such as anger from the liver, fear from the kidneys, and grief from the lungs. The Pericardium Meridian is also called the Heart Constrictor or Circulation-Sex Meridian.

Peak Hour of Function: Dog (7:00 to 9:00 p.m.)

---

[17] *Jue* (厥) is an older term for *Lao* (老) meaning "old." In more modern texts, "Old Yin" (老陰, Lao Yin) is used with these meridians. Chen Tuan uses the characters of 厥 (Jue) and 初 (Chu) as a compound to mean "the ending and beginning of things," and in the *Twenty-Four Dao Yin Seated Exercises* they indicate the ending of Old Yin Qi and the beginning of New Yang Qi. Hence, the idea of Old Yin Qi being *Faint* and New Yang Qi as being *Bright*. Chen Tuan's text uses the *Faint Yin Meridian* term to contrast with the previous *Bright Yang Meridian* designation.

Six Zi and the Twelve Primary Qi Meridians

Meridian Pathway: the Qi of this meridian flows down from the chest, through the arm, and ends in the tip of the middle finger. The meridian begins in the Qi point of *Celestial Pond* (天池, Tian Chi, P-1) and ends in *Central Rinse* (中冲, Zhong Chong, P-9).

This meridian begins in the middle of the chest, at the pericardium. It then flows over towards the armpit area, and then branches over descending internally through the diaphragm to the Upper, Middle, and Lower Triple Warmer Meridian, as it moves down the inside of the arm, through the middle of the wrist, and ending in the tip of the middle finger.

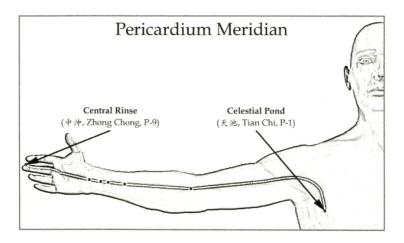

12. Faint Yin Foot (足厥陰, Zu Jue Yin) is connected with the vessels and cavities supporting the liver and so is called the Liver Meridian. It's governed by the elemental activities of Wood and is enjoined with the Gallbladder Meridian.

Official name: Minister of Replenishment.
Traditional name: Faint Yin Foot Liver Meridian.

Function: The liver is responsible for filtering, detoxifying, nourishing, replenishing, and storing blood; regulating the amount of blood circulation; withdrawing and storing blood during rest and sleep, and releasing it during physical movement and exercise.

Peak Hour of Function: Ox (1:00 to 3:00 a.m.)

Meridian Pathway: the Qi of this meridian flows upwards from the foot to the top of the head. This meridian begins in the Qi point of *Great Mound* (大敦, Da Dun, Lv-1) and ends in *Cyclic Door* (期門, Qi Men, Lv-14).

The Faint Yin Foot Meridian begins inside of the big toenail, crosses the top of the foot, passes in front of the inside ankle and up the inner aspect of the leg. It continues upward, passes the side of the knee, continues along the inner thigh to the groin and pubic region. From there it curves around the external genitalia and crosses the midline up to the lower abdomen, ending directly below the nipple.

Six Zi and the Twelve Primary Qi Meridians

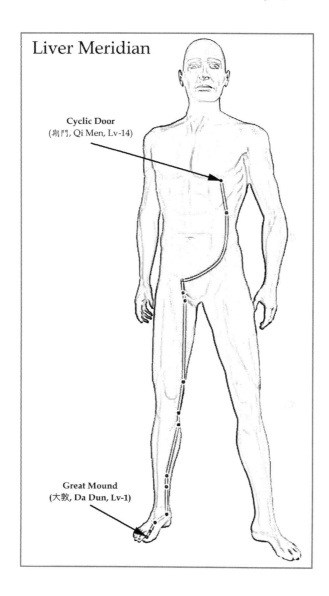

The Control and Function Meridians

In Medical Qigong the regulation of these two meridians is of the highest priority, as their fusion facilitates the Yin and Yang balance throughout the entire body. Even though they are described as two separate meridians, they are actually just one, representing the divisions of *Yang Fire* ascending (in the Dumai, 毒脈, Control Meridian, along the back of the body) and *Yin Essence* descending (in the Renmai, 任脈, Function Meridian, front of the body).

Circulating the Control and Function meridians is seen as fusing the elemental activities of Fire and Water. The Dumai is called the *Control Meridian* because it "controls" all the Yang meridians of the body, and the Renmai is called *Function Meridian* because it gives "function" to all the Yin meridians of the body.

The *Yang Fire* of the Control Meridian, in the Waidan perspective, begins at a Qi point at the tip of the tailbone vertebrae, called *Enduring Strength* (長強, Chang Qiang, Du-1) moves through the central pelvic area, then around the genitals (urethra in females and the penis in males). It then passes by the anus, and moves upwards inside the coccyx and sacrum, and then into the brain, where it moves to the lower end of the bridge of the nose and ends in the center of the upper gum of the mouth, at a Qi point called *Gum Crossing* (齦交, Yin Jiao, Du-28).

Six Zi and the Twelve Primary Qi Meridians

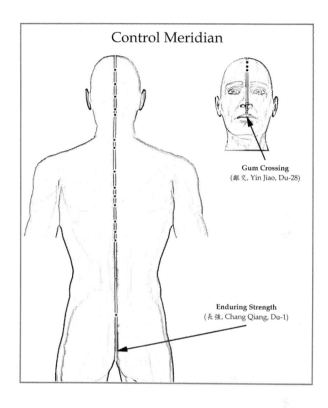

The *Yin Essence* of the Function Meridian, in the Waidan perspective, begins at a Qi point in the perineum, called *Converging Yin* (會陰, Hui Yin, Ren-1) moves through the pubic region through the center of the body, through the throat and up into the mouth to a Qi point called *Saliva Receiver* (承漿, Cheng Jiang, Ren-24).

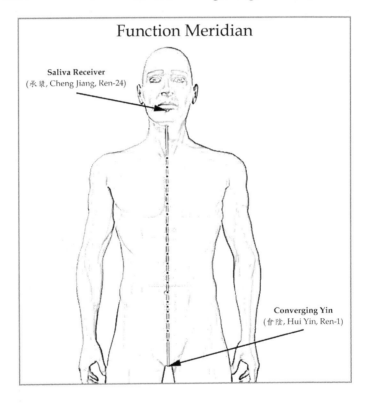

Six Zi and the Twelve Primary Qi Meridians

A brief note on the differences between the Waidan and Neidan perspectives on meridians: In Waidan, these two meridians, like the other twelve meridians, function on their external effects and correspondences with the Five Viscera, Six Bowels, the blood and Qi channels, and also within the muscles, sinews, and tendons of the body—meaning, their influence is considered as pertaining to physical and external functions of the body.

In the Neidan, or Internal Alchemy, aspects of there being Eight Extraordinary Qi Meridians, these are meridians that must be, in analogy, awakened in the body. They existed during the gestation period while in the womb, and for a short while after the birth and the severing of the umbilical cord, a division that is called in Taoism, Before Heaven (dwelling in the womb) and After Heaven (having left the womb).

There is a great difference in both the sensations, development, and regulations between External Qi meridians and cavities and those of the Internal Elixir meridians. See *Refining the Elixir* for more details on the Internal Alchemy meridians.

The Internal Organs and Functions

The following associations are taken from *The Yellow Emperor's Internal Medicine Classic* (黃帝內經, *Huang Di Nei Jing*), as Chen Tuan's instructions assume the reader has knowledge of these matters. In Chinese medicine, the term *Five Viscera* (五臟, Wu Zang), sometimes referred to as the Five Internal Organs (五內官, Wu Nei Guan, literally the *Five Inner Palaces*) applies to the liver, heart, lungs, kidneys, and Triple Warmer (spleen). The Five Viscera are the "solid" organs of the body, which connect to the Six Bowels (六腑, Liu Fu, or Six Entrails), the "hollow" organs of the body.

Five Viscera (五臟, Wu Zang)

Liver (Yang Organ, Wood Element): connected to the tear ducts. Controls the muscles of the body. Functions of the liver are controlled by the **Faint Yin Foot Liver Meridian.**

Heart (Yang Organ, Fire Element): connected to sweat glands. Controls the blood pulses of the body. Functions of the heart are controlled by the **Young Yin Hand Heart Meridian** and the **Faint Yin Hand Pericardium Meridian.**

Spleen (Central Organ, Half Yin/Half Yang, Earth Element): connected to the saliva glands. Controls the flesh of the body. Functions of the spleen are controlled by the **Ultimate Yin Foot Spleen Meridian.**

Lungs (Yin Organ, Metal Element): connected to the mucus membranes. Controls the skin of the body. Functions of the lungs are controlled by the **Ultimate Yin Hand Lung Meridian.**

Kidneys (Yin Organ, Water Element): connected to the sexual secretions. Controls the bones and marrow of the body. Functions of the kidneys are controlled by the **Young Yin Foot Kidney Meridian.**

Six Bowels (六腑, Liu Fu)

These six "hollow" organs represent the six divisions of the gastrointestinal tract, responsible for the removal, or evacuation, functions of the body.

Stomach (胃, Wei): The stomach is an expandable muscular organ, a tube between the esophagus and small intestine, located on the left side above the abdomen. Food first enters the stomach, and through the secretion of acids and enzymes the food is broken down for digestion. Stomach muscles contract periodically for the purpose of

The Internal Organs and Functions

churning the food for greater digestion, and to aid in delivering the liquified mixture to the small intestine.

The functions of the stomach are controlled by the **Bright Yang Foot Stomach Meridian.**

Small Intestine (小腸, Xiao Chang): The main function of the small intestine is the absorption of nutrients and minerals from the food we ingest. Ninety percent of the digestion and absorption of food occurs within the small intestine, the other ten percent takes place in the stomach and large intestine. The small intestine is about ten feet in length and maintains three main sections: duodenum (top), jejunum (left side), and ileum (right side).

The functions of the small intestine are controlled by the **Ultimate Yang Hand Small Intestine Meridian.**

Large Intestine (大腸, Da Chang): usually just referred to as the colon, this bowel is the final section of the gastrointestinal tract that absorbs water and vitamins, and converts digested food into feces. It is called large intestine because it is considerably thicker than the small intestine, but only about five feet in length. The large intestine is wrapped around the abdominal cavity, from the right side (ascending colon) it moves up across the top of the abdomen (transverse colon) and then down the left side (descending colon), which then connects with the rectum and anus.

The functions of the large intestine are controlled by the **Bright Yang Hand Large Intestine Meridian.**

Urinary Bladder (膀胱, Pang Guang): The urinary bladder is a sac located in the pelvic area behind and above the pubic bone. Urine is produced in the kidneys, but sent to the urinary bladder via two tubes called ureters, where the urine is then stored until it is evacuated through the urethra.

The functions of the urinary bladder are controlled by the **Ultimate Yang Foot Urinary Bladder Meridian.**

Gallbladder (膽, Dan): a small organ, but extremely important, that stores bile produced in the liver and helps in the digestion of fats in food in the duodenum of the small intestine. It is situated on the right side of the stomach just above the top portion of the large intestine. If the large intestine does not function properly, the bile it is storing may crystalize, creating gallstones which can become very painful and even life threatening if becoming infected.

The functions of the gallbladder are controlled by the **Young Yang Foot Gallbladder Meridian.**

Triple Warmer (三焦, San Jiao): the passageways for heat and fluids through the body. The Triple Warmer, not being an actual physical organ, rather an ethereal one, is divided into Upper, Middle, and Lower sections of the body. The classification of the Triple Warmer is the subject of a great deal of controversy even within Chinese medicine. The confusion comes from whether or not the definition is given by the Physicians (醫家, Yi Jia) or Taoist (道人, Dao Ren) practitioners of Chinese medicine. The Physicians list the Triple Warmer Hand (手三焦, Shou San Jiao) as being associated with the Pericardium Meridian, and the Triple Warmer Foot (足三焦, Zu San Jiao) with the Gallbladder Meridian. Taoists, however, don't view it solely as a meridian *per se*, but deem it as both a non-physical Production Organ and Removal Organ simultaneously, as it is considered a general metabolizer of ingested nutrients for the entire gastrointestinal tract. In some cases, Taoists include the spleen organ as part of the Triple Warmer in their lists. In this work, Chen Tuan takes the Taoist view of the Triple Warmer as an organ.

The functions of the Triple Warmer are controlled by the **Young Yang Hand Triple Warmer Meridian.**

Elemental Activities

During the twenty-four periods within a year certain natural responses (or elemental activities) are triggered within the body. These conditions are expressed as one of the Six Qi, or when out of balance, as one of the Six Excesses.

Six Qi (六氣) represent the six conditions of climate: *cold, wind, heat, moisture, fire,* and *drought*. In human physiology, these are the conditions of *coldness, airs, heat, dampness, fire,* and *dryness,* and it is one or more of these conditions that can cause illness and disease in the body if becoming extreme. The *Twenty-Four Dao Yin Seated Exercises* are designed to regulate these conditions.

Six Excesses (六淫, Liu Yin) are six conditions that can equally be applied to climate as well as to a person's physical and mental conditions. Excessive eating, excessive sexual dissipation, excessive emotions, or excessive toiling of the body can all bring about illness and disease. A common Chinese expression used when determining another person's mental state is to ask, "How's your weather?" Meaning, are you cold (distant), windy (scattered), hot (angry), damp (depressed), bright (cheerful), or dry (indifferent) in your temperament?

Chen Tuan's exercises and regimes are meant to ensure that these responses do not become excessive and thus create various illnesses. The cures and remedies listed in each of the *Twenty-Four Dao Yin Seated Exercises* are designed to ensure that the negative effects of the Six Excesses do not occur, which in Chinese medicine are termed as Yin or Yang deficiencies that can be applied to any of the Five Viscera, Six Bowels, meridians, or Qi points.

1. *Dry Metal* (燥金, Zao Jin): excessive dryness associated with the lungs.
2. *Cold Water* (寒水, Han Shui): excessive coldness associated with the kidneys.
3. *Wind Wood* (風木, Feng Mu): excessive wind associated with the liver.
4. *Ruling Fire* (君火, Jun Huo): excessive heat associated with the heart.
5. *Damp Earth* (濕土, Shi Du): excessive dampness associated with the spleen.
6. *Parched Earth* (渴土, Jue Tu): excessive aridness associated with the Triple Warmer.

Note that the element of Earth is indicated twice with *Damp Earth* and *Parched Earth*. This coincides with the correlation of the Earth element with the extended seasons of Late Summer and Long Summer, and as being a harmonized integration of Yin and Yang.

In the following diagram of the Six Zi's relationships to the Six Qi, note that there are two forms of Fire within the Six Qi. This Qi of *Secondary Fire* is explained in the following section.

Elemental Activities

The Six Zi Responding with the Six Qi Diagram[18]

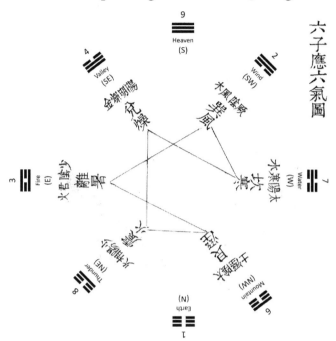

7) ☵ *Ultimate Yang*—**Cold Water** (太陽寒水, Tai Yang Han Shui) is represented by the trigram for Water (坎, Kan), Coldness (寒, Han) and the West (西, Xi).

2) ☴ *Faint Yin*—**Wind Wood** (厥陰風木, Jue Yin Feng Mu) is represented by the trigram for Wind (巽, Sun), Winds (風, Feng), and the Southwest (西南, Xi Nan).

---

18   From *A Collection on the Essentials of the Rivers He and Luo* (河洛精蘊, *He Lou Jing Yun*). Four volumes, early Qing dynasty work (reprinted by White Cloud Monastery, 1989).

3) ☲ *Young Yin*—**Fire Heat** (少陰離暑, Shao Yang Li Shu) is represented by the trigram for Fire (離, Li), Heat (暑, Shu), and the East (東, Dong).

6) ☷ *Ultimate Yin*—**Damp Earth** (太陰濕土, Tai Yin Shi Du) is represented by the trigram for Mountain (艮, Gen), Moisture (濕, Shi), and the Northwest (西北, Xi Bei).

8) ☳ *Young Yang*—**Secondary Fire** (少陽相火, Shao Yang Xiang Huo) is represented by the trigram Thunder (震, Zhen), Fire (火, Huo), and the Northeast (東北, Dong Bei).

4) ☱ *Bright Yang*—**Dry Metal** (陽明燥金, Yang Ming Zao Jin) is represented by the trigram for Valley (兌, Dui), Drought (燥, Zao), and the Southeast (東南, Dong Nan).

9) ☰ **Control Meridian** (毒脈, Du Mai) and 1) ☷ **Function Meridian** (任脈, Ren Mai) are represented by the trigrams Heaven (乾, Qian, South, 南, Nan) and Earth (坤, Kun, North, 北, Bei) respectively, and are rulers over the Six Zi and Six Qi. They are the foundations from which the Twelve Primary Meridians are classified as either a Yang or Yin meridian, or as a Hand (Yang/Heaven) or Foot (Yin/Earth) meridian.

Elemental Activities

Secondary Fire

The first elemental activity mentioned in Chen Tuan's Dao Yin exercises is *Secondary Fire* (相火, Xiang Huo). It occurs during the spring and autumn months. This term actually means a secondary form of heat (炁, Qi)[19] in the body; namely, heat produced in the lower body, the heat of sexual passion, and what is called "Formless Heat" in Internal Alchemy. This type of heat is a biological response that occurs during the middle of the first month of spring and throughout the beginning month of autumn. If this heat becomes too excessive it can adversely affect the internal organs.

This subject of sexual heat is an important aspect of Taoist cultivation, but is often cloaked, clouded, or covertly inserted into the texts. Generally speaking, Taoist writings and teachings prior to Zhang Daoling's reorganizing of Taoism into a religion[20] considered sexual energy practices,

---

[19] The common form of Qi (氣) applies to body temperature and what brings warmth to the body, whereas *Secondary Fire* is the type of heat (炁, Qi) developed from sexual passion. See *Refining the Elixir* for a fuller definition of these terms.

[20] Zhang Daoling (張道陵, 34–156 CE) is credited with turning Taoism from an unstructured philosophical teaching to an organized religious sect. His new religion was first called Five Pecks of Rice Sect (五斗米道, Wu Dou Mi Dao), as that was the fee for admission. Later it became the Celestial Masters Sect (天師派, Tian Shi Pai). This sect of Taoism still exists under the name of the Orthodox One (正一, Zheng Yi) and is headquartered at Dragon Tiger Mountain (龍虎山) in Jiangxi province.

at least in terms of their restorative and transformational aspects, as being crucial to an adept's cultivation for longevity and immortality. In chapter 15 of the *Master Who Embraces Simplicity*,[21] Ge Hong responds to a question about how a cultivator of internal arts can avoid illnesses:

> In doing everything possible to nourish your life, take the Immortal Medicines.[22] Also never tire of circulating your breaths.[23] Morning and night perform the calisthenics[24] for circulating your blood and Qi, so that they do not stagnate. You must practice sexual activity in the proper manner and time.[25] Eat and drink moderately, avoid drafts and dampness, and do not concern yourself over things

---

[21] Ge Hong's classical work, *Master Who Embraces Simplicity* (抱朴子, *Bao Pu Zi,* 320 CE), is one of Taoism's most important texts.

[22] *Immortal Medicines* can refer to metallurgical and herbal compounds as well as undertaking the processes (called medicines) of Reverting the Jing, Qi, and Shen into an Internal Elixir. See *Refining the Elixir* for more information.

[23] *Mobilizing the Qi* (運氣, Yun Qi).

[24] *Dao Yin* (導引) and *Tu Na* (吐呐) regimes.

[25] Taoist sexual practices include *Harmonizing the Yin and Yang* (和陰陽, He Yin Yang), *Refining Rosy Clouds* (煉霞, Lian Xia), *Rain and Clouds* (雨雲, Yu Yun), *Tigress and Dragon* (龍虎, Long Hu), along with many other teachings and practices. See *Daoist Sexual Arts: A Guide for Attaining Health, Youthfulness, Vitality, and Awakening the Spirit* (Valley Spirit Arts, 2015) for more information.

not of your endowments. Do all these things and you will never fall ill.

Like Ge Hong, many influential Taoist figures, such as Zhang Sanfeng, Lu Dongbin, He Xianggu, and others, advocated the use of Sexual Alchemy teachings (sexual practices) as a basis for advancing the processes of Internal Alchemy.

Li Qingyun, the 250-Year-Old Man, advised to engage in sexual activity according to the natural changes in nature. The idea of *Refining Rosy Clouds* means to regulate sexual activity in the seasons of spring and summer when the Qi is naturally in its *Sprouting* and *Growth* stages. In autumn and winter, as the Qi moves into the *Harvesting* and *Storage* periods (see the *Classifications of Qi* section), one should abstain from sexual activity.

The Jade Tablet Decrees on Nature and Life teaches sexual self-stimulation for the purpose of enhancing Jing energy within the kidneys. This practice of dual cultivation (because it is making use of self-stimulated sexual energy along with contemplative/visualization methods) is promoted to help in the process of Reverting Jing to Restore the Brain, a precursor for forming the Elixir of Immortality.

Rain and Clouds, a teaching originating with the Yellow Emperor that appears in the *Plain Girl Classic* (素女經, *Su Nu Jing)*, relies greatly on the idea that males should lessen and control ejaculation and females reduce and control menstrual flow so as to conserve Jing.

Within the sexual cultivation teachings of *Tigress and Dragon*, males make use of the *Yin to enhance the Yang* and females the use of *Yang to enhance the Yin* for achieving states of Spiritual Illumination through the practice of *Embracing the One* (抱一, Bao Yi).

In all Taoist sexual teachings, the common denominator lies within the idea of "conservation" along with "correct stimulation" so as not to cause any of the Five Elements, or activities of them, to become excessive. When males ejaculate too frequently, their Jing is diminished and damaged, especially concerning the functions of the lungs and kidneys, When the Jing is damaged, the Qi cannot accumulate, and if the Qi cannot be accumulated, the Shen can neither be retained nor attracted. It is the same with females, except the Jing is damaged by excessive and heavy menstruation, which adversely affects the functioning of the heart and kidneys.

On the other hand, through balancing and regulating the conservation and stimulation of sexual energy, we strengthen the activities and functions of the Five Elements (Wood, Fire, Earth, Metal, Water) and associated organs.

My teacher masterfully summarized all Taoist sexual arts in the following statement, *"Stimulation is far greater than dissipation."* Adding that as long people maintain sexual vitality, they can stay healthy, achieve longevity, and accomplish immortality. Conversely, when losing sexual vitality, they find old age, sickness, and death.

Use of Herbs and Foods

Within *The Book of Immortal Longevity of Ten Thousand Years,* Chen Tuan includes a section on the *Forty-Eight Medicinal Kung.* Each Kung offers herbal, plant, and/or mineral formulas that are best for curing a variety of specific illnesses. Listing all of them here would have been far too lengthy, and not completely germane to this work, but you'll find two of the Medicinal Kung at the back of this work: *The Venerable Sovereign Li Playing the Lute Pose,* along with the herbal formula Iron Date Pills, and *Xu Shenweng's Method for Preserving the Qi and Opening the Passes,* with the herbal formula Protecting Harmony Pills. I hope to publish a work on all *Forty-Eight Medicinal Kung* in a future volume.

The subject of herbs and foods in Taoism is paramount to self-cultivation, but not all Taoists follow the same path. Some Taoists are full-time vegetarians, for example, and some are not, while others may fast or abstain from eating meat on specific days of the month.

Li Qingyun, who was primarily vegetarian, would eat meat on certain occasions, but when doing so, he would sliver the meat and use it more as a seasoning than a main course. Eating heavy pieces of meat is hard on the stomach, small intestine, and large intestine, taking a great deal of energy for the bowels to digest. Being an herbalist, Li Qingyun strongly held the view that health, longevity, and immortality could not be maintained or achieved without herbs.

Li Qingyun advocated that certain herbs must be taken on a daily basis to achieve good health and longevity, and most certainly when cultivating immortality. He highly recommended taking He Shou Wu (何首烏), Huang Jing (黃精), Ling Zhi (苓芝), Ginseng (人蔘), and Goji berries (狗記).

On a regular basis, my teacher, who lived to 102, ate what he called *Immortal Soup*—a mixture of chestnuts, lotus seeds, dates, tofu, and ginseng, all boiled together to form a soup. He was also mostly vegetarian, and would often take one small cup (saki cup size) of an herbal brandy containing Deer Antler powder and ginseng each evening before bed, and especially during autumn and winter months.

Chen Tuan likewise recommends taking different herbs and foods appropriate to each season to keep the associated organ in good health. As he says, "There is excellent reason for this." The *Jade Tablet Decree on Nature and Life* confirms that no one can become immortal unless the Five Viscera are functioning in optimum health, and this occurs by performing the proper daily exercises and regimens and ingesting the proper herbs and foods.

Setting aside the principle that one needs to take herbs and eat foods suitable to a given season, there is also nothing fixed about the foods to be ingested. The main idea is to eat what is in season and the foods indigenous to the region in which you are living. Herbal formulas and medicinal prescriptions, then, are supplementary to this idea. Interestingly, macrobiotics developed its teachings with this core idea in mind.

In a humorous story that, I think, perfectly captures this section on food and herbs, a student once asked my teacher a very long and drawn out question on what he would eat in his daily routine to promote his development of Qi. Master Liang, appearing very serious, remained silent for a while, then said, "If I don't eat, I will die."

In the end, food is essential to our existence and we must eat to maintain body warmth, and equally to provide nutrition for the Five Viscera and to keep the Six Bowels functioning properly.

Preliminary Instructions

Breathing Methods and Regimes

Natural Breathing (自息, Zi Xi)

The two main breathing methods used in the exercises are Natural Breathing and Embryonic Breathing (or Reverse Breathing). The first rule of Natural Breathing is just that, to be "natural." Do not force the breath to be either long or deep. Let this happen naturally through practice. When inhaling, the abdomen expands, and it contracts during the exhalation. Each breath is inspired and expired through the nose with the tip of the tongue placed on the upper portion of the inside of the mouth. Natural Breathing is accomplished simply by putting all of your attention into the lower abdomen (Dan Tian) so that there is no forcing of the breath to be deep and slow.

Embryonic Breathing (胎息, Tai Xi)

The basic idea of performing Embryonic Breathing correctly is to contract the abdomen when inhaling and expand it when exhaling—the exact opposite of Natural Breathing. With Embryonic Breathing, imagine your abdomen is like a balloon and, in analogy, something squeezes the balloon causing the upper portion of the balloon to rise and expand. When doing so, roll the eyes upwards as if to gaze at the upper brain area, the tongue is held against the upper palate, and when inhaling draw the slightly. These are the physiological aspects of internally raising the energy in the body. Psychologically, the mind imagines and visualizes the energy rising from the lower abdomen up into the brain. In these respects, Embryonic Breathing is simple, but to get rid of the sensations of forcing and overextending the inhalation is much more difficult. Embryonic breathing is the preferred method with the *Four Season Qigong* exercises.

Closing the Breath (閉氣, Bi Qi)
Closing, or *Holding*, the Breath is sometimes called Tortoise Breathing (龜息, Gui Xi). With this "closing" method, the Qi concentrates in the area of attention, and when the breath is opened again, the Qi (and blood) rushes into that area of attention. Holding the breath is an expedient means for stimulating the Qi in certain cases. In Internal Alchemy, this method has a much more defined and frequent use.

Swallowing Nine Breaths (嚥九息, Yan Jiu Xi)
In Dao Yin, two types of regimes call for swallowing. One is the swallowing of saliva and the other for the swallowing of Qi (breath), or, more accurately, "ingesting Qi" (吸收氣, xi shou Qi). Initially, the swallowing of nine mouthfuls of breath/Qi is purely imaginary, as with each inhalation, you imagine the mouth fills with Qi and is then swallowed down just like when swallowing saliva. Over time, the air in the mouth will begin to feel more substantial when swallowing.

Preliminary Instructions

The practice of ingesting Qi begins with inhaling (through the nose) and visualizing the Qi as a white cloudy substance filling the mouth. Then swallow it while exhaling, visualizing and sensing it descending into the lower Elixir Field (abdomen). Repeat the process nine times. The use of ingesting Qi occurs in the *Four Season Qigong* exercises, not in the *Twenty-Four Dao Yin Seated Exercises,* as they accentuate the practice of swallowing saliva.

Swallowing the Saliva (嚥 液, Yan Ye)

This practice is the same exercise as *Rousing, Rinsing,* and *Swallowing* in Eight Brocades. The main function and purpose is to refine the "essence" (精, jing).

In *Rousing,* the tongue is made to circle in both clockwise and counterclockwise directions thirty-six times each way.

For *Rinsing,* the accumulated saliva is sucked back and forth across the tongue thirty-six times.

Lastly, to perform *Swallowing,* the hands are raised up to ear level, held in the fashion of "grasping the hands firmly." With the palms facing forward, suspend the head slightly upward and feel as though the nose is contracted inwards. Then divide the saliva by a third and with a slight force, swallow. When doing so, feel as though swallowing from the Mysterious Well (玄井, Xuan Jing) cavity (the center of the clavicle bone beneath the throat). Sense the saliva passing through the solar plexus and then into the lower Elixir Field. Perform two more actions of swallowing the saliva.

Circulating Mouthfuls of Qi (運氣口, Yun Qi Kou)

As in the process of swallowing Qi or saliva, the visualization of the Qi being a white cloudy substance is the same. The difference is that the Qi/breath in the mouth is visualized as revolving around the tongue as it is placed up against the upper palate. In Chinese medicine, the tongue is considered as the small spine of the body, with the underside of the tongue equating to the back of the body, and the topside of the tongue equating to the front of the body.

As in circulating the Qi up the actual spine and down the front of the body through the Dumai (毒脈) and Renmai (任脈) meridians, the Qi in the mouth is visualized in this method as moving up along the underside of the tongue and then down the topside. In this way the Qi is mobilized in a micro fashion as to what is done with the Renmai and Dumai meridians along the spine and front of the body.[26]

The use of Yun Qi Kou occurs in the Sleeping Kung and Medicinal Kung regimes, with slight variations in each exercise.

---

[26] With the tongue on the upper palate, it is like a person sitting in the mouth looking into the body, not facing out.

Knocking the Teeth (叩齒, Kou Chi)

In Eight Brocades Seated Qigong,[27] Li Qingyun says that knocking the teeth "collects the spirit." The main function is to stimulate the shen (神, spirit). When knocking the teeth, pay attention to the sensations heard and felt in both "Ear Gates" (耳門, Er Men). Position the back of the hands by each knee in a fist-like deportment, with the middle fingers of each hand slightly pressing into the centers of the palms—the *Dragon Cavity* (龍穴, Long Xue) is in the center of the left palm and the *Tiger Cavity* (虎穴, Hu Xue) is in the center of the right palm. This hand deportment is called "grasping the hands firmly."

Blowing-Out and Drawing-In (吐納, Tu Na)

This literally means to exhale and spit out the unclean air *(Tu)* and inhaling to take in clean air *(Na)*. The main function is to gather the "vital energy" (Qi). In practice this means to inhale through the nose (Na) into the lower Elixir Field (Dan Tian) and then with pursed lips exhale by blowing out (Tu). The palms of the hands are positioned over each ear, in a cupping-like fashion, so to block off external noises and allow the breath to be heard purely internally.

---

[27] See *The Immortal: True Accounts of the 250-Year-Old Man, Li Qingyun* and the companion work, *Li Qingyun: Longevity Methods of a 250-Year-Old Taoist Immortal* (Valley Spirit Arts, 2016) for information about the Eight Brocades Seated Qigong Exercises.

Breathing Patterns in the Exercises

Whether using Natural or Embryonic Breathing, the usual pattern is to inhale when turning the head, arm, or body to the indicated side and exhale when returning to the starting position, then repeating the inhaling and exhaling pattern on the other side. For some exercises, the inhale can be to one side and the exhale to the other, such as inhaling and turning the head to the left and exhaling while turning the head all the way to the right side. Sometimes it is just a matter of personal preference whether you want to take two cycles of Qi to complete both sides of a method, or to complete the movements in one cycle.[28]

The *Spring Kung, Summer Kung, Late Summer Kung,* and the first twelve *Dao Yin* exercises all start with the idea of working the left (Yang) side of the body, meridian, or method first, and then repeating on the right side.

The *Long Summer Kung, Autumn Kung, Winter Kung,* and *Dao Yin* exercises 13 through 24, reverse the pattern and work the right (Yin) side of the body, meridian, or method first, and then repeat with the left side.

---

[28] A *cycle of Qi* means taking one full breath of an inhale and exhale.

Preliminary Instructions

Massaging Qi Centers and Meridians

Just as the back of the body is considered Yang and the front is Yin, the left side of the body is Yang and the right side is Yin, and, as mentioned in the section on the Twelve Meridians, the hands are Yang and the feet are Yin.

With the *Twenty-Four Seated Dao Yin Exercises,* the Six Hand Meridians are associated with the six lunar months of spring and summer. They are further divided by having the Six Yang Hand Meridians related to spring, and the Six Yin Hand Meridians with summer. The Six Foot Meridians relate to the six lunar months of autumn and winter, with the Six Yang Foot Meridians in autumn and the Six Yin Foot Meridians in winter.

In the *Four Season Qigong* exercises, however, the meridians to be massaged relate to the organ of the season and the Five Viscera. Interestingly, these are all Yin Hand and Foot Meridians.

When the instructions say to massage a certain meridian, choosing which side branch of the meridian to massage first is not based on the meridian's Yin or Yang classification (such as Yang meridians starting or ending on the left side of the body and the Yin meridians as being associated with the right side). Since each meridian runs bilaterally on both sides of the body, the question remains on which side to massage, or which side to massage first.

In the exercises, massage both the left- and right-side branches of the designated meridian, but rather than looking at its Yin or Yang classification to determine which side to massage first, you accord with the season instead.

Just like with the Breathing Patterns, this means that for spring and summer (the Yang half of the year), you massage the left-side branch of each Yin or Yang meridian first, then complete it on the right side.

In autumn and winter (Yin half of the year), reverse the pattern and massage the right-side branch first, then the left side. This principle applies to all the *Four Season Qigong* and *Twenty-Four Seated Dao Yin Exercises.*

Daily Practice Advice

The secret to mastering anything in life is through repetition. When we repeat things they become part-and-parcel to our actions and from that we experience a freedom, a freedom from anxiety and apprehension about the action or task at hand.

Ideally, both of Chen Tuan's yearly regimes would be practiced each day, but it's also fine to just practice one of the regimes and forego the other. In fact, these two exercise systems are rarely shown together in the older Chinese texts.

If you are serious about Setting Up the Foundation for Internal Alchemy, however, then you should practice both regimes diligently for at least one full year, keeping the following advice in mind:

- Morning and evening perform the specific kung for the season, including massaging the indicated meridian of the regime.

- At least once per day, perform the indicated Dao Yin Seated Exercise, along with rubbing the Qi points and massaging the designated meridian of that exercise.

- Each morning ingest the recommended herbs for the season.

- Each noon hour eat the suggested foods for nourishing, strengthening, and repairing the specific organ for the season.

- Sit in meditation once or twice a day, even if for just fifteen minutes. The Qi in the body can't move freely unless there is some sense of calmness and stillness in the body and mind.

As stated in the Preface, the exercises in this book are for Setting Up the Foundation of Internal Alchemy. Without doing the work of a caterpillar forming its cocoon, it can never turn into a butterfly. Without doing the work of restoring your Three Treasures of Jing, Qi, and Shen, you will never have the necessary components (cocoon if you will) to transform into an immortal. These exercises can help you on your path, whether you simply want to find moments of peace and calm within your day, improve your health and well-being, or take on the work of immortalizing your spirit, *Chen Tuan's Four Season Internal Kung Fu* will take you far along the way.

Spring

Spring Kung
春功

Season of Birth for Repairing, Nourishing, and Strengthening the Liver

Green Dragon
青龍

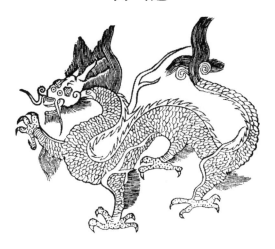

The celestial Green Dragon represents the eastern quadrant of the Heavens and the elemental activities of Wood. On the terrestrial level, the liver is symbolically represented by an Earthly Dragon of whitish and brown color.

Chen Tuan's Four Season Internal Kungfu

The Three Hexagrams Ruling the Spring Months

	#24	#19	#11	#34	#43	#1	#44	#33	#12	#20	#23	#2
	Fu	Lin	Tai	Da Zhuang	Guai	Qian	Gou	Dun	Pi	Guan	Bo	Kun
Earthly Branch	子	丑	寅	卯	辰	巳	午	未	申	酉	戌	亥
	Zi	Chou	Yin	Mao	Chen	Si	Wu	Wei	Shen	You	Xu	Hai
Twelve Animals	Rat	Ox	Tiger	Rabbit	Dragon	Snake	Horse	Goat	Monkey	Rooster	Dog	Pig
Month	11	12	1	2	3	4	5	6	7	8	9	10
Hour	23-1	1-3	3-5	5-7	7-9	9-11	11-13	13-15	15-17	17-19	19-21	21-23

First Moon	Second Moon	Third Moon
#11	#34	#43
Tai	Da Zhuang	Guai
Peacefulness	*Great Strength*	*Decision*

Animal Sign

Tiger	Rabbit	Dragon

Earthly Branch

Yin (寅)	Mao (卯)	Chen (辰)

Liver, 肝, Gan

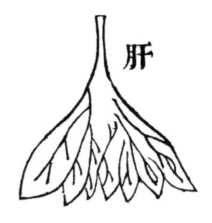

The liver is the mother of the heart and son of the kidneys. The liver is the viscera which maintains the status of leader of all the other viscera. It is symbolized as a dragon and its spirit name is *Dragon Mist* (龍烟, Long Yan), and is designated as *Embracing Brightness* (含明, Han Ming).

The shape of the liver is that of a dragon, resembling a hanging bottle gourd of a white and brown color. Its right side has four lobes and the left has three. The liver is located in the upper right-hand portion of the abdominal cavity, beneath the diaphragm and on top of the stomach, right kidney, and intestines.

The liver stores the Heavenly Spirit (魂, Hun). At night (during unconscious states) the Hun resides in the liver, and during the day (in conscious states) it resides on the top of the head.

The Qi pulse for the liver emerges in *Great Mound* (大敦, Da Dun, Lv-1, inside of the big toenail).

Comments

The liver is the largest gland in the human body and its function is to keep the body pure of toxins and other harmful substances. The liver produces bile, and the salts in the bile, as well as the following functions:
1. Breaks up the fats from the foods we eat into smaller particles so that the small intestines can more easily absorb and process them.
2. Detoxifies the blood from harmful substances, like drugs and alcohol, introduced into the body.
3. Stores a certain level of vitamins and iron.
4. Converts stored sugar to functional sugars when glucose levels drop below normal.
5. Breaks down hemoglobin, insulin, and various hormones.
6. Converts ammonia to urea, a vital process for the metabolism.
7. Disposes old red blood cells.

In Chinese medicine, good liver function is paramount to good health, as anything either absorbed by the skin, breathed into the body, or ingested will have to be processed by the liver. Even the chemicals in the water we shower or bathe with will be absorbed and processed by the liver. The liver is also the only organ of the body that will regenerate itself after being injured, such as a perforated liver from alcohol or drug abuse. An unhealthy liver does not convert ammonia into urea, and therefore either the breath or urine will have an ammonia odor to it, which is one of the meanings in these texts about the "removing of foul airs." Because the liver is the mother of the heart, a bad or dysfunctional liver can cause heart ailments, and the liver, being the son of the kidneys, will be adversely affected if the kidneys are failing in their functions.

In Taoism, a requisite for obtaining immortality involves gaining optimum health of the Five Viscera (liver, heart, lungs, kidneys, and spleen), which in turn brings good health to the Six Bowels (small intestine, large intestine, urinary bladder, gallbladder, stomach, and Triple Warmer). The liver must be restored and protected so that all the other organs and functions can be in good health.

In reading about Taoists wandering into the high mountains to live within nature, the reason wasn't just about cultivating in a peaceful setting. It equally had to do with being in an environment where they could inhale fresh mountain air, drink clean mountain water, and ingest potent herbs, and all this to have a profound effect on the liver.

This idea of being in nature is clearly represented in Chen Tuan's springtime instructions, as they are associated with the color green (for restoration, like being in nature), the element of Wood (trees and being outdoors), and a dragon, the symbol of Yang energy. The repair and restoration of the liver to a Taoist cultivating Internal Alchemy is paramount to attaining good health, longevity, and immortality.

Green Dragon Kung

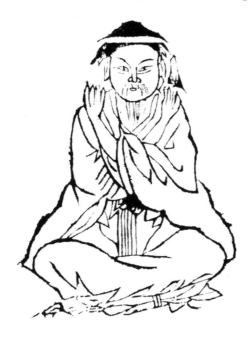

In springtime the body is changing from extreme Yin into Yang. The Protective Qi[29] that encompasses the body and guards it from acquiring disease is growing during this period. Because the spirit is heightened at this time, the emotions also run high, so it's helpful to employ deep gentle breathing to bring calmness to the mind. As

---

[29] *Protective Qi* (保氣, Bao Qi) is a Chinese term referring to having a highly functional bodily immune system along with the mental state of being in good spirits.

Chen Tuan's Four Season Internal Kungfu

the liver is associated with the Wood element, it's more beneficial to make use of the Fire element during this time. Wood is produced by Water, and Wood produces Fire.

This kung, performed for repairing, nourishing, and strengthening the liver during the three months of spring, involves first sitting cross-legged [facing east],[30] with the two palms alternately resting on each shoulder [left arm in front of the right].

Knock the teeth three times; close the breath [閉氣, Bi Qi] and breathe[31] in [through the nose] nine times [making nine short inhalations while holding the breath], and then exhale slowly.

Next, make sure the body is facing south[32] and breathe in nine mouthfuls and swallow nine times [嚥九息, Yan Jiu Xi].

Then equally and alternately press the two hands slowly into the shoulders. First press the right hand in and then the left, doing so to each side three times.

---

[30] Each exercise will indicate to start facing the direction of the associated animal, but this isn't mandatory. However, whichever direction you are facing at the start, the instructions will have you turn the body to face south at some point.

[31] Embryonic Breathing is recommended for the entire exercise. See *Preliminary Instructions* p. 75. Note that Chen Tuan advises to let the exhalation be longer than the inhalation in this kung.

[32] Here the direction of the exercise changes to face south. Turn your whole body and cross the hands and arms again.

Spring

Next, interlock the fingers of both hands. Then with the back of the hands held firmly against the chest, turn the palms and wrists over fifteen times.[33]

After having driven out the corrupt air, sit with the eyes fixed and eyelids slightly closed, puff out the breath slowly, little by little.[34]

The cure [of the liver] is complete when the face becomes flushed and tears begin to flow.

This kung cures obstructions of the liver stemming from harmful winds and corrupted airs[35] and so prevents diseases from developing in the liver.

These exercises must be performed each morning and evening during the spring months, without missing even one day.[36] With a determined heart the repair and nourishment of the liver will be complete.

---

[33] Keep the hands attached to the chest as they rotate in and out.

[34] Slowly exhale to "exhaust one breath." Build up to exhaling for at least twelve heartbeats, but don't strain to do this. Eventually, you will be able to slowly exhale for longer periods.

[35] "Harmful winds" (惡風, E Feng) and "corrupted airs" (貪氣, Tan Qi) not only applies to breathing in polluted toxic air, but also can refer to the ill effects of negative or extreme emotional responses that cause the breath and Qi to become corrupted and irregular.

[36] Chen Tuan doesn't repeat this instruction about when to practice in the other three seasonal Qigong regimes, but they should be practiced twice daily as well. The routine carries throughout the entire year, but the methods change with each of the four seasons.

If using Embryonic Breathing, let the exhalation be somewhat longer than the inhalation. Rub the area of the liver on the back several times, and then massage the path of the liver meridian with vigorous action.[37]

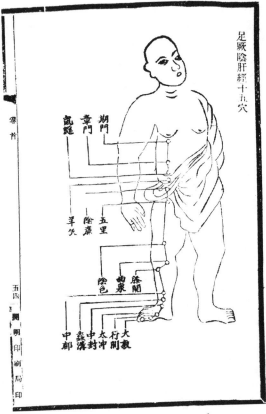

Faint Yin Foot Liver Meridian

---

37   See *Preliminary Instructions*, p. 81. In spring, massage the meridian path along the left foot and leg first, then the right.

Herbs for Cleansing and Nourishing the Liver

The following herbs and foods are recommended because they remove metals and toxins from the liver and help repair a damaged liver.

Milk Thistle [水飛薊, Shui Fei Ji]

Improves the function of the liver. Daily dosage: 12 to 15 grams per day.

Chinese Red Dates [紅棗, Hong Zao, Jujube]

Protects the liver. Daily dosage: 5 to 10 pieces per day.

Turmeric [鬱金, Yu Jin]

Stimulates the Liver Meridian, removes toxins from the liver, and repairs a damaged liver. Daily dosage: 3 to 9 grams per day.

Turmeric is a plant of the ginger family grown in southern regions of China and India. In India, turmeric is one of the Seven Vedic Healing Plants.

Foods for Expelling Foul Airs (Detoxing) of the Liver

In spring, it is best to consume food and drinks that are essentially green and from leafy plants and vegetables.

Green Teas [綠茶, Lu Cha]

All green teas are high in antioxidants and so have a very cleansing effect on the liver. High doses of green teas are not good for the liver, so one or two cups of green tea per day is sufficient and beneficial.

Green Leaf Vegetables [綠色葉菜, Lu Se Ye Cai]

The most effective are gai lan (芥蘭), bitter gourd, arugula, dandelion greens, spinach greens, and mustard greens. Baby kale is beneficial, but not adult kale. Adult kale absorbs a great deal of metals before harvesting and so can be harmful to the liver.

Soy Paste [味噌, Wei Seng, Miso] with Roasted Seaweed [紫菜, Zi Cai, Nori] as Soup [湯, Tang]

Miso soup is an excellent mixture for eliminating the metals the liver absorbs from various foods and toxins. This is an especially good soup for anyone undergoing chemotherapy or radiation treatments for cancer, and specifically those with liver cancer. One bowl of the soup per day is sufficient, unless undergoing cancer treatment, then two bowls per day is recommended.

The Six Dao Yin Seated Exercises of Spring

First Spring Exercise

立春正月節

Spring Begins—First Moon

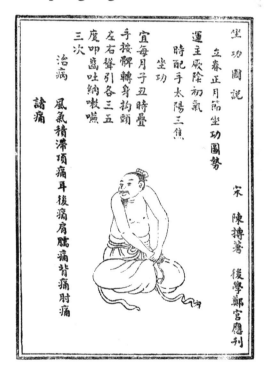

Dao Yin Exercise 1

Chen Tuan's Four Season Internal Kungfu

Month: First Moon
Days: 1st thru 14th
Hours: Zi (子) 11:00 p.m. to 1:00 a.m.
Chou (丑) 1:00 to 3:00 a.m.

坐功
Seated Exercise

運主厥陰初氣
Mobilize and control the Faint Yin to initiate New Qi.

Faint Yin is referencing the organs and Qi of the liver and pericardium. Through the exercise, *New Yang Qi* is being stimulated to control the effects of the old Faint Yin Qi acquired during the winter months. Faint Yin Qi is controlled in the first period of this month by initiating Ultimate Yang Qi and stimulating the Qi of the Triple Warmer.

時配手太陽三焦
At this time enjoin the Ultimate Yang Hand Meridian and the Triple Warmer.[38]

On the left side of the body, rub the areas of the beginning and end points of the Small Intestine Meridian 36 times in a clockwise manner. Start with *Young Marsh* (少澤, Shao Ze, SI-1) and finish with *Listening Palace* (聽宮, Ting Gong, SI-19).

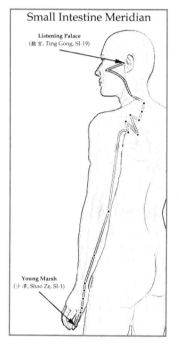

Next, vigorously massage the left-side pathway of the *Ultimate Yang Hand Meridian* three times. Repeat on the right side of the body, first rubbing the Qi points and then massaging the meridian path three times.

---

38 The Small Intestine and Triple Warmer meridians run close to each other, so naturally massaging one of them will affect the other.

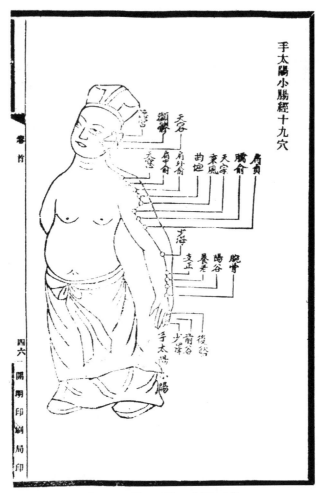

*Ultimate Yang Hand Meridian
of the Small Intestine, 19 Qi Points*

Spring

治病
Medicinal Cure

Remedies rheumatism and blockages [from weak blood circulation and muscular tension] causing pain in the neck, shoulders, ears, back, elbows, and arms.

旨示
Instructions

Enfold the two hands, left over the right. Press the hands into the left thigh. Turn the body and twist the neck to the left and then to the right, 15 times to each side.

終功
Concluding Kung

Knock the Teeth [叩齒, Kou Chi] 36 times; perform 24 Blowing-Out and Drawing-In [吐納, Tu Na] breaths, and Swallow the Saliva [嚥液, Yan Ye] three times.

Second Spring Exercise

雨水正月中

Rain Waters—Middle of First Moon

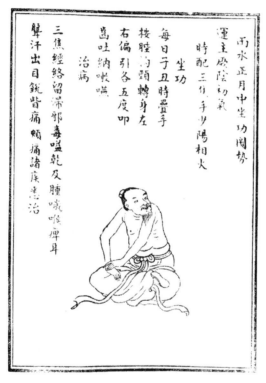

Dao Yin Exercise 2

Month: 1st Moon
Days: 15th thru 30th
Hours: Zi (子) 11:00 p.m. to 1:00 a.m.
Chou (丑) 1:00 to 3:00 a.m.

坐 功
Seated Exercise

運主厥陰初氣
Mobilize and control the Faint Yin to initiate New Qi.

Faint Yin is referencing the organs and Qi of the liver and pericardium. Through the exercise, *New Yang Qi* is being stimulated to overcome the effects of the old Faint Yin Qi acquired during the winter months. Faint Yin Qi is controlled in the second period of this month by stimulating the Qi and the Young Yang Hand Triple Warmer Meridian.

Spring

時配三焦手少陽相火
At this time enjoin the Young Yang Hand Meridian of the Triple Warmer.

The Triple Warmer meridian begins in the Qi point of *Pass Rinse* (關沖, Guan Chong, SJ-1) and ends in the *Silk Bamboo Opening* (絲竹空, Si Zhu Kong, SJ-23).

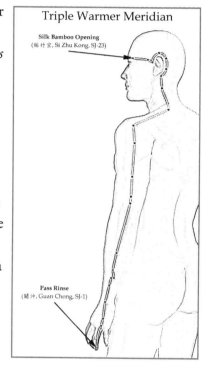

On the left side of the body, rub the area of these two points 36 times in a clockwise manner, starting with *Pass Rinse* and finishing with *Silk Bamboo Opening*.

Next, vigorously massage the pathway of the Young Yang Hand Meridian three times. Repeat on the right side of the body.

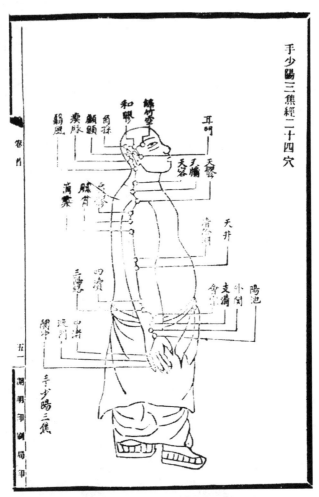

*Young Yang Hand Meridian
of the Triple Warmer, 24 Qi Points*

相火
Secondary Fire

At this time of year the Qi of the Triple Warmer (Fire) naturally creates Secondary Fire. It is too strong because of an excess of Qi in the Young Yang Hand Triple Warmer Meridian, and so must be regulated and brought into harmony. The exercise is designed to help alleviate this excess.

If the heat of sexual desire becomes too strong, rub the middle of the soles of the feet, the *Bubbling Well* (湧泉, Yong Quan) Qi cavities, with the thumbs.

治病
Medicinal Cure

Remedies difficulties in swallowing, deafness, eye pain, and eliminates obstructions and accumulation of noxious energies [such as reflux symptoms] throughout the three divisions of the esophagus [throat, chest, and stomach areas].

旨示
Instructions

Enfold the two hands, left over right. Press the hands into the right thigh. Turn the body and twist the neck left and right, alternating 15 times to each side.

Chen Tuan's Four Season Internal Kungfu

終功
Concluding Kung

Knock the Teeth [叩齒, Kou Chi] 36 times; perform 24 Blowing-Out and Drawing-In [吐納, Tu Na] breaths, and Swallow the Saliva [嚥液, Yan Ye] three times.

Third Spring Exercise

驚蟄二月節

Waking Insects—Second Moon

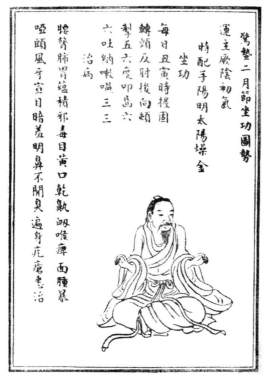

Dao Yin Exercise 3

Month: 2nd Moon
Days: 1st thru 14th
Hours: Chou (丑) 1:00 to 3:00 a.m.
Yin (寅) 3:00 to 5:00 a.m.

坐功
Seated Exercise

運主少陽二氣
Mobilize and control the Two Qi of Young Yang.

Young Yang is referencing the organs and Qi of the Triple Warmer and gallbladder. *Mobilizing and controlling the Two Qi* of Young Yang is initiated by the regime of *Closing the Fists Firmly*, where the middle fingers of each hand press into the Dragon (left-hand palm) and Tiger (right-hand palm) cavities.

時配手陽明大腸燥金
At this time enjoin the Bright Yang Hand Meridian of the Large Intestine.

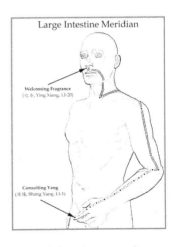

The meridian begins in the Qi point of *Consulting Yang* (商陽, Shang Yang, LI-1) and ends in *Welcoming Fragrance* (迎香, Ying Xiang, LI-20). On the left side of the body, rub the areas of these two points 36 times in a clockwise manner, starting with *Consulting Yang* and finishing with

Welcoming Fragrance. Next, vigorously massage the pathways of the Bright Yang Hand Meridian three times. Repeat on the right side of the body.

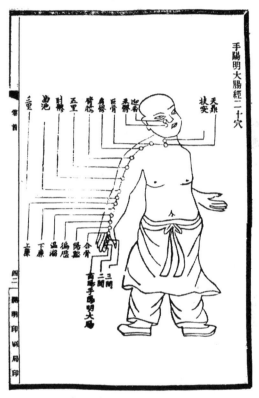

*Bright Yang[39] Hand Meridian
of the Large Intestine, 20 Qi Points*

---

[39] Some older texts may call this meridian *Bright Purity* (清明, Qing Ming) instead of *Bright Yang* (陽明, Yang Ming). They may use *Bright Purity* to indicate the hand meridian and *Bright Yang* to indicate the foot meridian, but these are the same and are both *Bright Yang*.

燥金
Dry Metal

At this time of year the lungs (Metal) naturally experience an excess of dryness because the Qi of the Bright Yang Hand Meridian is insufficient. The exercise alleviates this problem.

Dry Metal can also occur from excessive seminal or menstrual dissipation.

治病
Medicinal Cure

Remedies problems associated with the loins and lower back, and pains of the lungs and stomach. Cures dry mouth, yellowing of the eyes, headaches, toothache, darkened vision, sensitivity to light, decreased sense of smell, and boils anywhere on the body.

Spring

旨示
Instructions

Close the fists firmly. Turn the head while moving the elbows like wings [of a bird], drawing the arms forward then backward, doing so 30 times.⁴⁰

終功
Concluding Kung

Knock the Teeth [叩齒, Kou Chi] 36 times; perform 24 Blowing-Out and Drawing-In [吐納, Tu Na] breaths, and Swallow the Saliva [嚥液, Yan Ye] three times.

---

40 With the elbows tucked in and the fists facing upward, the arms are held at 45 degree angles from the body. As you inhale and turn the head to the left, flip the arms (wings) over so that the fists face each other in front of the chest, palms facing down. Exhale and turn the head back to the front while extending the fists forward, dropping the elbows so that the palms face up again. The arms are sticking straight out from the body held at shoulder level with the fists shoulder-width apart and in line with each other. The idea is to move your arms outward away from the body during the inhale and exhale (one cycle of Qi).

To return to the starting position and complete one repetition, inhale and turn the head to the right side, while flipping the arms over and drawing them back so that the fists face each other again. Exhale and turn the head to face forward while flipping the arms into their starting positions.

The outward flipping of the arms and drawing them back is completed in two cycles of Qi and counts as one rep. Repeat the entire series of movements 29 more times.

Fourth Spring Exercise

春分二月中

Spring Equinox—Middle of Second Moon

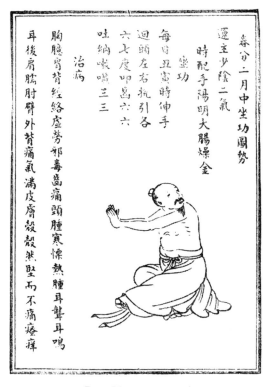

Dao Yin Exercise 4

Month: 2nd Moon
Days: 15th thru 29th
Hours: Chou (丑) 1:00 to 3:00 a.m.
　　　　　Yin (寅) 3:00 to 5:00 a.m.

Chen Tuan's Four Season Internal Kungfu

坐功
Seated Exercise

運主少陽二氣
Mobilize and control the Two Qi of the Young Yin.

Young Yin is referencing the organ and Qi of the heart and kidneys. *Mobilizing and controlling the Two Qi* of Young Yin is initiated by the alternating movements of the hands while turning the head. Turning left is the Dragon Qi, and turning right is the Tiger Qi.

時配手陽明大腸燥金
At this time enjoin the Bright Yang Hand Meridian of the Large Intestine.

The meridian begins in the Qi point of *Consulting Yang* (商陽, Shang Yang, LI-1) and ends in *Welcoming Fragrance* (迎香, Ying Xiang, LI-20). On the left side of the body, rub the areas of these two points 36 times in a clockwise manner, 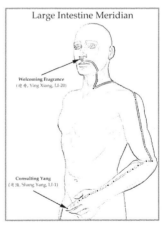 starting with *Consulting Yang* and finishing with *Welcoming Fragrance*.

Next, vigorously massage the pathway of the Bright Yang Hand Meridian three times. Repeat on the right side of the body.

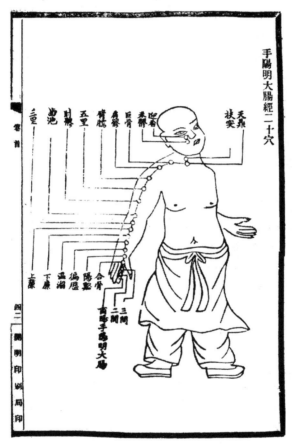

*Bright Yang Hand Meridian
of the Large Intestine, 20 Qi Points*

燥金
Dry Metal

At this time of year the lungs (Metal) naturally experience an excess of dryness because the Qi of the Bright Yang Hand Large Intestine Meridian is insufficient. The exercise alleviates this problem.

Dryness in the lungs can also be exasperated from excessive seminal or menstrual dissipation.

治病
Medicinal Cure

Remedies coldness and weakness by removing noxious air from the chest, shoulders, and back. Stimulates the capillaries of the body. Relieves toothaches, fevers, difficulties in hearing, and earaches. Use when having pain in the shoulder, elbows, upper arm, and back.

旨示
Instructions[41]

Extend the left leg and position both arms to the right diagonal [holding them at chest level—see the exercise illustration]. Turn the head left and right 42 times. Repeat to the other

---

[41] The text instructions say to perform this exercise in a low squatting position. If this is too difficult, you can practice it in a sitting posture, as you do in the second part of Exercise 19. See p. 230.

side, switching the leg and arm positions, and turning the head left and right 42 times.[42]

終功
Concluding Kung

Knock the Teeth [叩齒, Kou Chi] 36 times; perform 24 Blowing-Out and Drawing-In [吐納, Tu Na] breaths, and Swallow the Saliva [嚥液, Yan Ye] three times.

---

[42] Because of the numerous head turns, this exercise is a good example for choosing to breathe in one Qi cycle while turning the head to the left and right. See *Preliminary Instructions,* p. 80.

Fifth Spring Exercise

清明三月節

Bright Purity—Third Moon

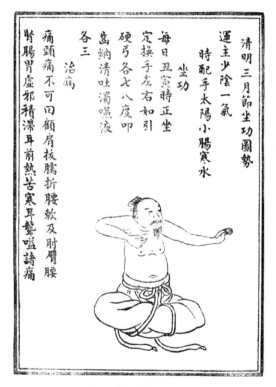

Dao Yin Exercise 5

Month: 3rd Moon
Days: 1st thru 14th
Hours: Chou (丑) 1:00 to 3:00 a.m.
　　　　　Yin (寅) 3:00 to 5:00 a.m.

Chen Tuan's Four Season Internal Kungfu

坐功
Seated Exercise

運主少陰二氣
Mobilize and control the Two Qi of Young Yin.

Young Yin is referencing the organ and Qi of the heart and kidneys. *Mobilizing and controlling the Two Qi* of Young Yin is initiated by the alternating movements of the hands while turning the head. Turning left is the Dragon Qi, and turning right is the Tiger Qi.

時配手太陽小腸寒水
At this time enjoin the Ultimate Yang Hand Meridian of the Small Intestine.

The meridian begins in the Qi point of *Young Marsh* (少澤, Shao Ze, SI-1) and ends in *Listening Palace* (聽宮, Ting Gong, SI-19). On the left side of the body, rub the areas of these two points 36 times in a clockwise manner, starting with *Young Marsh* and finishing with *Listening Palace*.

Next, vigorously massage the pathway of the Ultimate

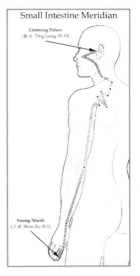

Spring

Yang Hand Meridian three times. Repeat on the right side of the body.

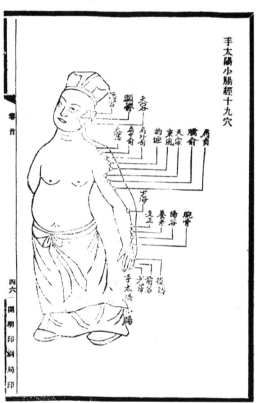

Ultimate Yang Hand Meridian of the Small Intestine, 19 Qi Points

寒水
Cold Water

At this time of year the kidneys (Water) naturally experience an excess of coldness because the Qi of the Ultimate Yang Hand Small Intestine Meridian is insufficient. The exercise alleviates this problem.

治病
Medicinal Cure

Remedies weakness and noxious airs of the loins, kidneys, intestines, and stomach. Also remedies painful swallowing, pain in the ears, pain and stiffness of the neck, and pain in the shoulders, arms, and thighs.

旨示
Instructions

Sit upright. Alternate the hands left and right as though drawing a bow 56 times.[43]

終功
Concluding Kung

Knock the Teeth [叩齒, Kou Chi] 36 times; perform 24 Blowing-Out and Drawing-In [吐納, Tu Na] breaths, and Swallow the Saliva [嚥液, Yan Ye] three times.

---

[43] Inhale and extend the arms to the left side, exhale as you draw in the imaginary bow string with your right hand (this is one cycle of Qi). Inhale while turning your extended left arm across the body to the right side and extend the right arm to the right side. Exhale as you now draw in the bow string with your left hand (one cycle of Qi). Repeat these movements, alternating one cycle of Qi to each side a total of 56 times.

Sixth Spring Exercise

穀雨三月中

Corn Rain—Middle of Third Moon

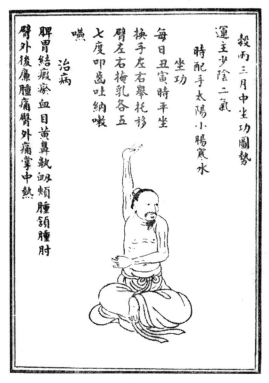

Dao Yin Exercise 6

Month: Third Moon
Days: 15th thru 30th
Hours: Chou (丑) 1:00 to 3:00 a.m.
Yin (寅) 3:00 to 5:00 a.m.

Chen Tuan's Four Season Internal Kungfu

坐 功
Seated Exercise

運主少陰二氣
Mobilize and control the Two Qi of Young Yin.

Young Yin is referencing the organ and Qi of the heart and kidneys. *Mobilizing and controlling the Two Qi* of Young Yin is initiated by the alternating movements of raising the hands. The left is the Dragon Qi, and the right is the Tiger Qi.

時配手太陽小腸寒水
At this time enjoin the Ultimate Yang Hand Meridian of the Small Intestine.

The meridian begins in the Qi point of *Young Marsh* (少澤, Shao Ze, SI-1) and ends in *Listening Palace* (聽宮, Ting Gong, SI-19). On the left side of the body, rub the areas of these two points 36 times in a clockwise manner, starting with *Young Marsh* and finishing with *Listening Palace*.

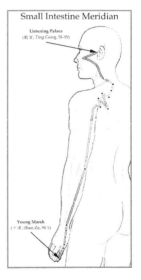

Spring

Next, vigorously massage the pathway of the Ultimate Yang Hand Meridian three times. Repeat on the right side of the body.

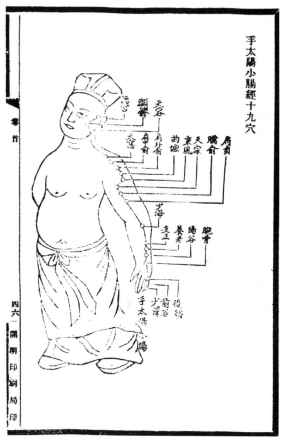

Ultimate Yang Hand Meridian of the Small Intestine, 19 Qi Points

Chen Tuan's Four Season Internal Kungfu

寒水
Cold Water

At this time of year the kidneys (Water) naturally experience an excess of coldness because the Qi of the Ultimate Yang Hand Meridian is insufficient. The exercise alleviates this problem.

治病
Medicinal Cure

Remedies and removes blood obstructions in the spleen and stomach, treats yellowness in the eyes, nose bleeds, and stimulates blood in the cheeks, neck, and arms.

旨示
Instructions

Sit upright and alternately raise the left and right arms as though supporting something above. When raising the left hand, bring the right hand to cover the left breast, and vice versa, doing so 35 times with each arm.

終功
Concluding Kung

Knock the Teeth [叩齒, Kou Chi] 36 times; perform 24 Blowing-Out and Drawing-In [吐納, Tu Na] breaths, and Swallow the Saliva [嚥液, Yan Ye] three times.

Summer

Summer Kung
夏功

Season of Growth for Repairing, Nourishing, and Strengthening the Heart

Red Bird
朱雀

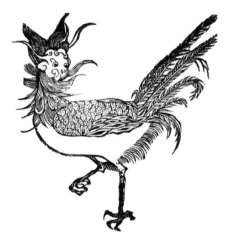

The celestial Red Bird represents the southern quadrant of the Heavens and the elemental activities of Fire. The terrestrial representation of the heart is symbolically represented by a phoenix.

Chen Tuan's Four Season Internal Kungfu

The Three Hexagrams Ruling the Summer Months

	#24	#19	#11	#34	#43	#1	#44	#33	#12	#20	#23	#2
	Fu	Lin	Tai	Da Zhuang	Guai	Qian	Gou	Dun	Pi	Guan	Bo	Kun
Earthly Branch	子 Zi	丑 Chou	寅 Yin	卯 Mao	辰 Chen	巳 Si	午 Wu	未 Wei	申 Shen	酉 You	戌 Xu	亥 Hai
Twelve Animals	Rat	Ox	Tiger	Rabbit	Dragon	Snake	Horse	Goat	Monkey	Rooster	Dog	Pig
Month	11	12	1	2	3	4	5	6	7	8	9	10
Hour	23-1	1-3	3-5	5-7	7-9	9-11	11-13	13-15	15-17	17-19	19-21	21-23

Fourth Moon	Fifth Moon	Sixth Moon
#1	#44	#33
Qian	Gou	Dun
Creativity of Heaven	*Pairing*	*Retreating*

Animal Sign

Snake	Horse	Goat

Earthly Branch

Si (巳)	Wu (午)	Wei (未)

Summer

Heart, 心, Xin

The heart is the son of the liver and mother of the spleen. It is sometimes called by its spirit name, *Red Ruler* (紅君, Hong Jun), as the heart is where the spirit is stored. Its official name is *Spirit Guard* (神尹, Shen Yin), and its personal name is *Divine Light* (靈光, Ling Guang). The heart organ resembles a scarlet bird with a dove's tail, and also looks like an upside down lotus flower.

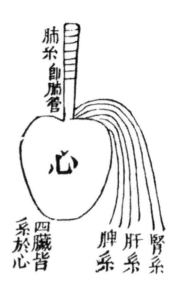

The heart is located just behind and slightly left of the breastbone.

The Qi pulse for the heart emerges from the chest at *Ultimate Well* (極泉, Ji Quan, H-1).

Comments

The heart is a muscular organ that is responsible for the pumping of blood through a network of arteries and veins called the cardiovascular system. The heart is located just behind and a little left of the breastbone, and is about the size of a person's fist. The heart is surrounded by a sac called the pericardium. There are four chambers that make up the heart:

1. The right atrium receives blood from the veins and then pumps it into the right ventricle.
2. The right ventricle receives blood from the right atrium, loaded with oxygen, and pumps it into the lungs.
3. The left atrium takes in oxygenated blood from the lungs and pumps it into the left ventricle.
4. The left ventricle, the real worker of the heart, pumps oxygen-rich blood into the entire body. There is also a web of nerve tissue that runs through the heart which issues a very complex signal system for the contracting and relaxing of the heart.

Red Bird Kung

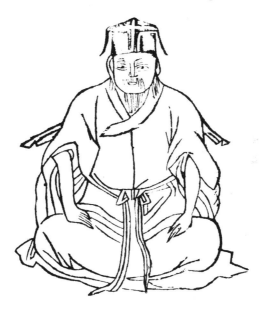

The body's Protective Qi is strengthened during this time and this aids in releasing excessive Qi retained by the internal organs. These summer exercises are meant to keep the heart in a proper state of Yin. The heart is associated with the Fire element. Therefore it is more beneficial to employ activities of the Earth element during this time.

The exercise is to be performed for repairing, nourishing, and strengthening the heart during the three months of summer [fourth, fifth, and sixth lunar months]. These exercises make pervious the Five Viscera, the Six Bowels, and the seven apertures of the heart.

The proper course for these exercises is to sit cross-legged [facing south], with both hands clenched into fists. Push down [with strength] into the left thigh and then the right, alternating 15 times with each hand [30 times total].

Next, raise the left hand as though lifting a bag of rice and supporting it over the head. Then do the same with the right hand. One time with each hand.

Then clasp both hands and place the bottom of the left foot within them and hold the breath [閉氣, Bi Qi] for at least the count of twelve heartbeats. Repeat with the right foot. Perform 15 times for each foot [30 times total]. This will drive out all diseases caused by harmful airs in the heart and thorax.

Next, close the eyes, swallow the saliva three times [嚥九息, Yan Jiu Xi], and knock the teeth three times. Afterwards make a *hem* sound [like clearing the throat]. This will cure any grief in the heart or ulcers in the mouth.

Facing south, breathe in nine mouthfuls and swallow nine times [嚥九息, Yan Jiu Xi].

To conclude, sitting upright, throw the fists forward [as if punching] and bring them back six times.

During the summer months the body is changing from a state of weak Yang to extreme Yang. The heart is a Yin organ, but Yin energy is lessened during the summer, which causes a heightened sense of emotions, and this can cause the heart to become excessively Yang.

These exercises open all seven apertures of the heart. Chinese medicine asserts that when all seven apertures are open there is high intelligence in the person. Those with a moderate intelligence, only five openings are pervious. Those who are intensely ignorant, all openings are obstructed, and no Qi can pass through.

If using Embryonic Breathing allow the inhalation to be longer than the exhalation so as to keep a calm mind and to aid in leading excessive Qi residing in the heart to move the lungs.

Rub the heart from the center outward a few times and then massage along the Heart and Pericardium meridians.[44] Do not dwell on the breath or directly upon the heart, as the Qi mobilizes to where the mind-intent [意, Yi] leads it, and doing so will cause the Qi to rise into the lungs and cause a dysfunction of the diaphragmatic membrane, as this membrane must descend when inhaling.

---

[44] Massage the left chest and arm first then the right. Both meridians will be affected at the same time as they run close to each other.

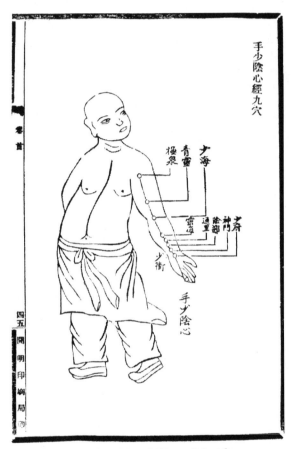

Young Yin Hand Heart Meridian

Summer

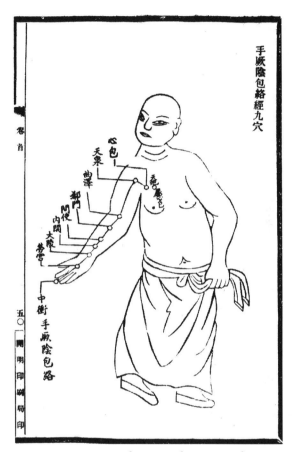

Faint Yin Hand Pericardium Meridian

Herbs for Nourishing the Heart

Hawthorn Fruit [山楂, Shan Zha]

Reduces fat cells and mucus accumulation, and improves blood flow. Using raw hawthorn helps eliminate blood stasis. Hawthorn fruit (usually powdered) is prescribed in Chinese medicine for blood problems in the spleen, stomach, and liver. Because of its enhanced effect on improving blood flow and reducing lipids (fat cells in the blood), it is highly recommended for nourishing the heart. Daily dosage: 10 to 15 grams.

Ginseng [人蔘, Ren Sen]

White American ginseng is best. Ginseng improves blood circulation to the heart and strengthens the immune system. Ginseng aids in the reduction of cholesterol and has shown positive effects on increasing the elasticity of blood vessels. Taoism considers it a longevity herb. Daily dosage: 30 to 50 grams.

Ginkgo Biloba [白果, Bai Guo]

Increases capillary circulation and expands blood vessels. Very good in treating cardiovascular diseases. These are the yellow seeds from the maidenhair tree (銀杏, yin xing). Daily dosage: 10 grams.

Dong Quai [當歸, Dong Gui]
Treats blockages in arteries and veins, and helps increase blood circulation. Especially good for women to aid in controlling and reducing menstrual flow. Also recommended for those suffering from diabetes. Daily dosage: 3 to 10 grams.

Foods for Expelling Foul Airs (Detoxing) of the Heart

Green Teas [綠茶, Lu Cha]
All green teas are high in antioxidants and so have a very cleansing effect on the heart. High doses of green teas are not good for the heart. Just one or two cups per day is sufficient and beneficial.

Pine Nuts [松仁, Song Ren]
Pine nuts contain a potent antioxidant called pycnogenol in its bark, needles, and nut that helps reduce inflammation in the blood vessels, lowering the risk of plaque buildup and so protects the heart from blood clotting. Daily dosage: best if taken in decoction, 10 to 15 grams.

Cinnamon [桂皮, Gui Pi and 肉皮, Rou Pi]
Gui Pi is the cinnamon leaves and Rou Pi is the bark. Cinnamon is very good for the heart and

promotes blood circulation and the lung Qi. Daily dosage: 3 to 10 grams.

Cinnamon is also considered in Chinese medicine as an excellent substance for counteracting effects of diabetes.

Ling Zhi [靈芝, Reishi]

The reishi mushroom (red reishi is best) has numerous benefits for all Five Organs, but is especially good for the heart and the immune system. If suffering from diabetes or hypertension, drink extra water after taking the mushroom to prevent producing too much oxalate. Reishi has also been found to help cure and prevent hepatitis B virus. Do not use in large amounts or for long-term periods (unless curing an illness). It's best if taken daily during the summer months, and periodically during other months. Daily dosage: 3 to 10 grams decocted in water.

The Six Dao Yin Seated Exercises of Summer

First Summer Exercise
立夏四月節
Summer Begins—Fourth Moon

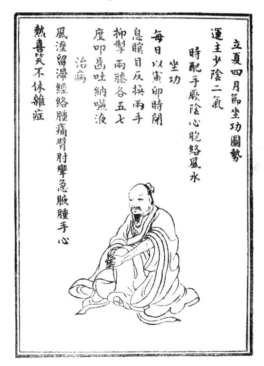

Dao Yin Exercise 7

Chen Tuan's Four Season Internal Kungfu

Month: Fourth Moon
Days: 1st thru 14th
Hours: Yin (寅) 3:00 to 5:00 a.m.
Mao (卯) 5:00 to 7:00 a.m.

坐功
Seated Exercise

運主少陰二氣
Mobilize and control the Two Qi of Young Yin.

Young Yin is referencing the organ and Qi of the heart and kidneys. *Mobilizing and controlling the Two Qi* of Young Yin is initiated by the movements of alternately pressing the knees. Pressing the left knee is stimulating the Dragon Qi, and pressing the right knee affects the Tiger Qi.

時配手厥陰心包絡風木
At this time enjoin the Faint Yin Hand Meridian of the Pericardium.

The meridian begins in the Qi point of *Celestial Pond* (天池, Tian Chi, P-1) and ends in *Central Rinse* (中沖, Zhong Chong, P-9).

On the left side of the body, rub the areas of these two points 24 times in a clockwise manner, starting with *Celestial Pond* and finishing with *Central Rinse*.

Summer

Next, vigorously massage the pathway of the Faint Yin Hand Meridian three times. Repeat on the right side of the body.

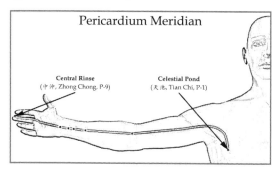

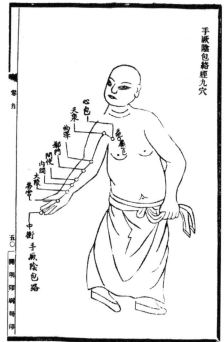

Faint Yin Hand Pericardium Meridian, 9 Qi Points

風木
Wind Wood

At this time of year the liver (Wood) experiences an excess of wind because the Qi of the Faint Yin Hand Pericardium Meridian is insufficient. The exercise alleviates this problem.

治病
Medicinal Cure

Remedies wind and dampness that collects in the Jing Luo [經絡], the blood vessel network of the arteries, veins, and capillaries, causing swollen and painful arms and armpits, and excessive heat in the palms of the hands.

旨示
Instructions

Close the breath [閉氣, Bi Qi] and darken the eyes. Inhale while turning the hands over and pressing the palms into the left knee. Exhale to starting position and repeat the movements 35 times before moving to the right knee.[45]

---

[45] Sitting, position the left knee in front of the body with the left foot flat on the ground. Interlock the hands, turn them outward, and place the back of the hands against the front of the left knee. Then inhale and rotate the hands to face the body. Exhale while flipping them back out. Maintain contact the whole time.

終功
Concluding Kung

Knock the Teeth [叩齒, Kou Chi] 36 times; perform 24 Blowing-Out and Drawing-In [吐納, Tu Na] breaths, and Swallow the Saliva [嚥液, Yan Ye] three times.

Second Summer Exercise
小滿四月中
Small Fullness—Middle of Fourth Moon

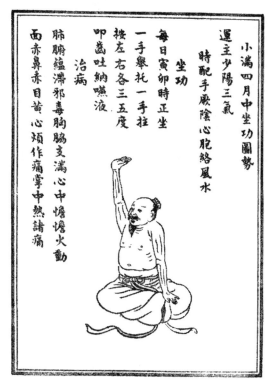

Dao Yin Exercise 8

Month: Fourth Moon
Days: 15th thru 30th
Hours: Yin (寅) 3:00 to 5:00 a.m.
Mao (卯) 5:00 to 7:00 a.m.

Chen Tuan's Four Season Internal Kungfu

坐功
Seated Exercise

運主少陽三氣
Mobilize and control the Three Qi of Young Yang.

Young Yang is a reference to the organ and Qi of the Triple Warmer (and gallbladder). Young Yang is associated with heat, so *mobilizing and controlling the Three Qi* of Young Yang is about stimulating the Three Qi, the three divisions of the Triple Warmer (Upper, Middle, and Lower), to bring heat to the Three Treasures of Jing, Qi, and Shen. The three divisions of the exercise—Raising, Supporting, and Pressing—are what affect the Upper, Middle, and Lower divisions of the Triple Warmer.

時配手厥陰心包絡風木
At this time enjoin the Faint Yin Hand Meridian of the Pericardium.

The meridian begins in the Qi point of *Celestial Pond* (天池, Tian Chi, P-1) and ends in *Central Rinse* (中沖, Zhong Chong, P-9). On the left side of the body, rub the areas of these two points 24 times in a clockwise manner, starting with *Celestial Pond* and finishing with *Central Rinse*. Next, vigorously massage the pathway of the Faint Yin Hand Meridian three times. Repeat on the right side of the body.

Summer

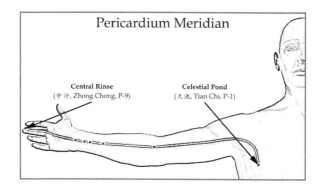

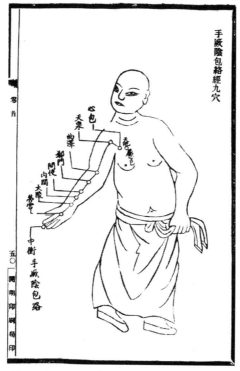

*Faint Yin Hand Pericardium Meridian,
9 Qi Points*

Chen Tuan's Four Season Internal Kungfu

風木
Wind Wood

At this time of year the liver (Wood) experiences an excess of wind because the Qi of the Faint Yin Hand Pericardium Meridian is insufficient. The exercise alleviates this problem.

治病
Medicinal Cure

Remedies obstructions in the liver and lungs, swelling in the thorax and ribs, flushing heat in the face, yellowish eyes, pain or fear in the heart, and overheated palms.

旨示
Instructions

Sit upright. Raise the left hand as if supporting something above and press the right hand on the right calf. Repeat on the other side, alternating left and right sides 12 times each side.

終功
Concluding Kung

Knock the Teeth [叩齒, Kou Chi] 36 times; perform 24 Blowing-Out and Drawing-In [吐納, Tu Na] breaths, and Swallow the Saliva [嚥液, Yan Ye] three times.

Third Summer Exercise

芒種五月節

Grain in Ear—Fifth Moon

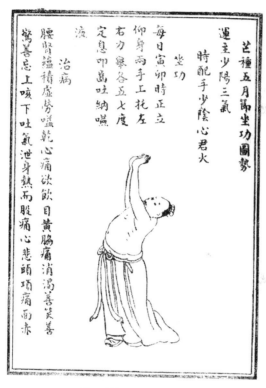

Dao Yin Exercise 9

Month: Fifth Moon
Days: 1st thru 14th
Hours: Chou (丑) 1:00 to 3:00 a.m.
Yin (寅) 3:00 to 5:00 a.m.

Chen Tuan's Four Season Internal Kungfu

坐功
Seated Exercise[46]

運主少陽三氣
Mobilize and control the Three Qi of Young Yang.

Young Yang is a reference to the organ and Qi of the Triple Warmer (and gallbladder). Young Yang is associated with heat, so *mobilizing and controlling the Three Qi* of Young Yang is about stimulating the Three Qi, the three divisions of the Triple Warmer (Upper, Middle, and Lower), to bring heat to the Three Treasures of Jing, Qi, and Shen. The three divisions of the exercise—Bending Back, Lifting, and Supporting—are what affect the Upper, Middle, and Lower divisions of the Triple Warmer. The three breaths used—inhaling, holding, and exhaling—also stimulate the Triple Warmer.

These stretches also aid in generating new blood and Qi to the gallbladder.

---

[46] Even though the text indicates this exercise as being seated, the instructions say to stand as this is better for stimulating the Jing/essence. Also, the exercise illustration shows the adept standing.

Summer

時配手少陰心君火
At this time enjoin the Young Yin Hand Meridian of the Heart.

The meridian begins in the Qi point of *Ultimate Well* (極泉, Ji Quan, H-1) and ends in *Little Rinse* (少沖, Shao Chong, H-9).

On the left side of the body, rub the areas of these two points 24 times in a clockwise manner, starting with *Ultimate Well* and finishing with *Little Rinse*.

Next, vigorously massage the pathway of the Young Yin Hand Meridian three times. Repeat on the right side of the body.

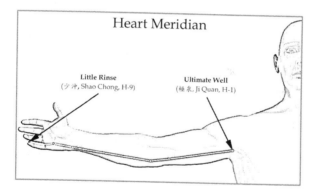

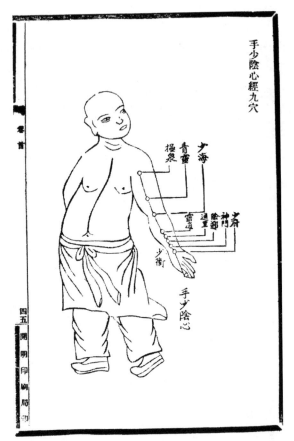

Young Yin Hand Heart Meridian, 9 Qi Points

君火
Ruling Fire

At this time of year the heart (Fire) naturally experiences an excess of heat because the Qi of the Young Yin Hand Heart Meridian is insufficient. The exercise alleviates this problem.

Summer

治病
Medicinal Cure

Remedies weakness in the loins and kidneys, dryness in swallowing, pain in the heart and ribs, yellow eye, thirst, excessive heat in the body, neck pain, redness in the face, cough and phlegm, diarrhea, excessive passage of wind, and controls [Jing] emission of semen [and reduction of menstrual flow in women].

旨示
Instructions

Standing, lean the body backwards while extending the arms upward. Feel as if exerting great strength to lift something heavy and then supporting it. Inhale when lifting up, close the breath [閉氣, Bi Qi] while supporting, and exhale when bringing the arms down [returning to the upright position]. Repeat 35 times.

終功
Concluding Kung

Knock the Teeth [叩齒, Kou Chi] 36 times; perform 24 Blowing-Out and Drawing-In [吐納, Tu Na] breaths, and Swallow the Saliva [嚥液, Yan Ye] three times.

Fourth Summer Exercise

夏至五月中

Summer Solstice—Middle of Fifth Moon

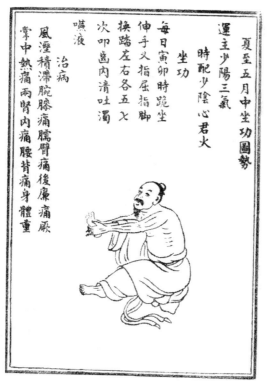

Dao Yin Exercise 10

Month: 5th Moon
Days: 15th thru 30th
Hours: Yin (寅) 3:00 to 5:00 a.m.
Mao (卯) 5:00 to 7:00 a.m.

坐功
Seated Exercise

運主少陽三氣
Mobilize and control the Three Qi of Young Yang.

> *Young Yang* is a reference to the organ and Qi of the Triple Warmer (and gallbladder). Young Yang is associated with heat, so *mobilizing and controlling the Three Qi* of Young Yang is about stimulating the Three Qi, the three divisions of the Triple Warmer (Upper, Middle, and Lower), to bring heat to the Three Treasures of Jing, Qi, and Shen. The three divisions of the exercise—Stretching, Interlocking, and Bending—are what affect the Upper, Middle, and Lower divisions of the Triple Warmer.

時配手少陰心君火
At this time enjoin the Young Yin Hand Meridian of the Heart.

> The meridian begins in the Qi point of *Ultimate Well* (極泉, Ji Quan, H-1) and ends in *Little Rinse* (少沖, Shao Chong, H-9). On the left side of the body, rub the areas of these two points 24 times in a clockwise manner, starting with *Ultimate Well* and finishing with *Little Rinse*. Next, vigorously massage the pathway of the Young Yin Hand Meridian three times. Repeat on the right side of the body.

Summer

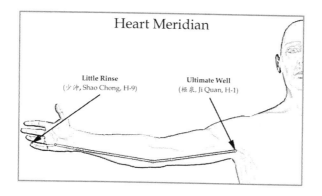

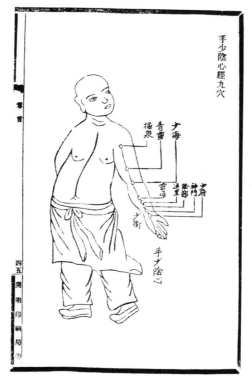

Young Yin Hand Heart Meridian, 9 Qi Points

君火
Ruling Fire
At this time of year the heart (Fire) experiences an excess of heat because the Qi of the Young Yin Hand Heart Meridian is insufficient. The exercise alleviates this problem.

治病
Medicinal Cure
Remedies obstructed breath [Wind] and stagnant dampness [rheumatism], pain in the knees, ankles, arms, kidneys, loins, spine, and feelings of heaviness in the body.

旨示
Instructions
In a seated or low squatting posture, stretch out the hands, interlock the fingers, and bend them over the bottom of the left foot. Perform 35 times and repeat with the right foot.[47]

---

[47] Draw in the foot toward the body after seizing it. It helps to perform Embryonic Breathing when inhaling and bending over to seize the foot. Exhale when drawing the foot in and bringing the hands back to their starting position in front of the chest.

終功
Concluding Kung

Knock the Teeth [叩齒, Kou Chi] 36 times; perform 24 Blowing-Out and Drawing-In [吐納, Tu Na] breaths, and Swallow the Saliva [嚥液, Yan Ye] three times.

Fifth Summer Exercise
小暑六月節
Lesser Heat—Sixth Moon

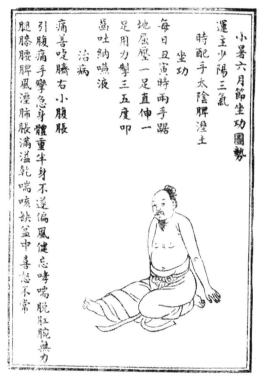

Dao Yin Exercise 11

Month: Sixth Moon
Days: 1st thru 14th
Hours: Chou (丑) 1:00 to 3:00 a.m.
Yin (寅) 3:00 to 5:00 a.m.

Chen Tuan's Four Season Internal Kungfu

坐功
Seated Exercise

運主少陽三氣
Mobilize and control the Three Qi of Young Yang.

Young Yang is a reference to the organ and Qi of the Triple Warmer (and gallbladder). Young Yang is associated with heat, so *mobilizing and controlling the Three Qi* of Young Yang is about stimulating the Three Qi, the three divisions of the Triple Warmer (Upper, Middle, and Lower), to bring heat to the Three Treasures of Jing, Qi, and Shen. The three divisions of the exercise—bending back and pressing the hands down, bending one leg inward, and stretching out the other leg—are what affect the Upper, Middle, and Lower divisions of the Triple Warmer.

時配手太陰肺濕土
At this time enjoin the Ultimate Yin Hand Meridian of the Lungs.

The meridian begins in the Qi point of *Central Mansion* (中府, Zhong Fu, Lu-1) and ends in *Young Consulter* (少商, Shao Shang, Lu-11). On the left side of the body, rub the areas of these two points 24 times in a clockwise manner, starting with *Central Mansion* and finishing with *Young Consulter*.

Summer

Next, vigorously massage the pathway of the Ultimate Yin Hand Meridian three times. Repeat on the right side of the body.

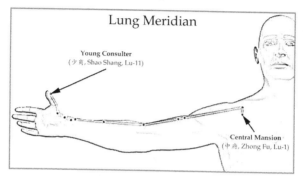

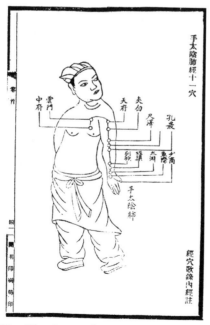

Ultimate Yin Hand Meridian of the Lungs, 11 Qi Points

濕土
Damp Earth

At this time of year the spleen (Earth) experiences an excess of dampness because the Qi of the Ultimate Yin Hand Meridian is insufficient. The exercise alleviates this problem.

治病
Medicinal Cure

Remedies rheumatism of the legs, knees, thighs, and loins. Relieves excessive phlegm in the lungs, asthma, cough, pain in the middle sternum, vicious sneezing, distended abdomen, arthritis, memory loss, heaviness of the body, whooping cough, weak wrists, and excessive emotions of joy and anger.

旨示
Instructions

Position the hands behind the body, pressing them flat on the ground, and bend the right foot under the body. Stretch out the left foot with strength [sliding it back on the exhale]. Perform 15 times, then repeat with the right foot.

終功
Concluding Kung

Knock the Teeth [叩齒, Kou Chi] 36 times; perform 24 Blowing-Out and Drawing-In [吐納, Tu Na] breaths, and Swallow the Saliva [嚥液, Yan Ye] three times.

Sixth Summer Exercise

大暑六月中

Greater Heat—Middle of Sixth Moon

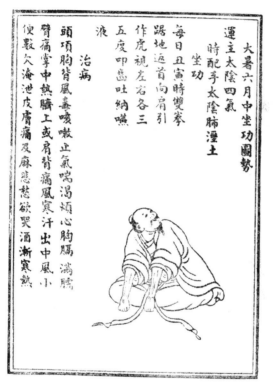

Dao Yin Exercise 12

Month: Sixth Moon
Days: 15th thru 30th
Hours: Chou (丑) 1:00 to 3:00 a.m.
Yin (寅) 3:00 to 5:00 a.m.

Chen Tuan's Four Season Internal Kungfu

坐功
Seated Exercise

運主太陰四氣
Mobilize and control the Four Qi of Ultimate Yin.

Ultimate Yin is a reference to the organs and Qi of the lungs and spleen. *Mobilizing and controlling the Four Qi* of Ultimate Yin is then associated with both Metal and Earth. Within this exercise Metal and Earth stimulate the Four Qi—lungs and large intestine (Metal), and spleen and Triple Warmer (Earth). The four divisions of the exercise—sitting in a heap, grasping the ground (Earth), rotating the head, and maintaining the countenance of a Tiger (Metal)—are what remedy the dampness of the spleen.

時配手太陰肺濕土
At this time enjoin the Ultimate Yin Hand Meridian of the Lungs.

The meridian begins in the Qi point of *Central Mansion* (中府, Zhong Fu, Lu-1) and ends in *Young Consulter* (少商, Shao Shang, Lu-11).
On the left side of the body, rub the areas of these two points 24 times in a clockwise manner, starting with *Central Mansion* and finishing with *Young Consulter*. Next, vigorously massage the pathway

Summer

of the Ultimate Yin Hand Meridian three times. Repeat on the right side of the body.

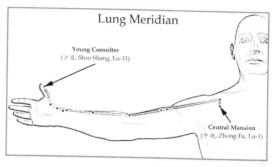

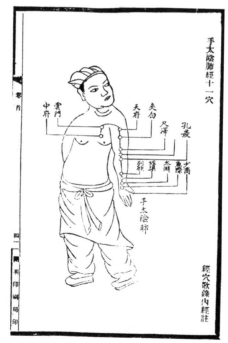

*Ultimate Yin Hand Meridian of the Lungs,
11 Qi Points*

濕土
Damp Earth

At this time of year the spleen (Earth) experiences an excess of dampness because the Qi of the Ultimate Yin Hand Spleen Meridian is insufficient. The exercise alleviates this problem.

治病
Medicinal Cure

Remedies rheumatism in the head, neck, chest, and back. Relieves cough, asthma, lack of thirst, fullness of the chest, arm pain, overheated palms, and pain above the navel, shoulders, and back. Remedies cold and hot perspiration, and excessive crying and feelings of grief.

旨示
Instructions

Sit like a heap on the ground [not a formal cross-legged posture, with the hands in fists touching the ground as if they were grasping the Earth] and alternately twist the head towards each shoulder. Using the countenance of a tiger, rotate the head 15 times to each side.

終功
Concluding Kung

Knock the Teeth [叩齒, Kou Chi] 36 times; perform 24 Blowing-Out and Drawing-In [吐納, Tu Na] breaths, and Swallow the Saliva [嚥液, Yan Ye] three times.

Late Summer and Long Summer Exercises

Season of Repairing, Nourishing, and Strengthening the Spleen

Yellow Dragon
黃 龍

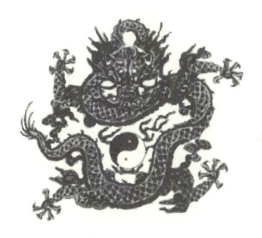

The celestial Yellow Dragon represents the center of the four quadrants of the Heavens and the elemental activities of Earth.

The following two additional exercises are not specifically designated as part of the Four Seasons, rather they are designed to compensate for the intermediate period between summer and autumn, termed *Late Summer* and *Long Summer*. The Late Summer Kung is performed during the second half of the sixth month and Long Summer is added to the first half of the seventh month. They are meant to augment the strengthening of the spleen and Triple Warmer. Both exercises drive away rheumatism that is obstructive to the spleen and aid in digestion through the Six Bowels.

Late Summer Kung
Extend the left foot while bringing down the hands to seize it. Draw in the foot, pulling it in with the hands. Extend the foot again, and draw it back. Do this 15 times, then repeat on the right side. Perform the exercise in the morning.

Long Summer Kung
In a kneeling position, both hands are positioned as though grasping the ground. Turn the head slowly, going to the right side first, then to the left side. Use an energy that looks like a Tiger intently gazing at prey. Do this 15 times. Perform in the evening.

Autumn

Autumn Kung
秋 功

*Season of Harvesting for Repairing,
Nourishing, and Strengthening the Lungs*

White Tiger
白 虎

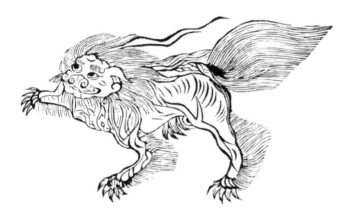

The celestial White Tiger represents the western quadrant of the Heavens and the elemental activities of Metal. The terrestrial animal representation for the lungs is the image of a crane.

Chen Tuan's Four Season Internal Kungfu

The Three Hexagrams Ruling the Autumn Months

	#24	#19	#11	#34	#43	#1	#44	#33	#12	#20	#23	#2
	Fu	Lin	Tai	Da Zhuang	Guai	Qian	Gou	Dun	Pi	Guan	Bo	Kun
Earthly Branch	子 Zi	丑 Chou	寅 Yin	卯 Mao	辰 Chen	巳 Si	午 Wu	未 Wei	申 Shen	酉 You	戌 Xu	亥 Hai
Twelve Animals	Rat	Ox	Tiger	Rabbit	Dragon	Snake	Horse	Goat	Monkey	Rooster	Dog	Pig
Month	11	12	1	2	3	4	5	6	7	8	9	10
Hour	23-1	1-3	3-5	5-7	7-9	9-11	11-13	13-15	15-17	17-19	19-21	21-23

Seventh Moon	Eighth Moon	Ninth Moon
#12	#20	#23
Pi	Guan	Bo
Adversity	*Contemplation*	*Removing*

Animal Sign

Monkey	Rooster	Dog

Earthly Branch

Shen (申)	You (酉)	Xu (戌)

Lungs, 肺, Fei

The lungs are the son of the spleen and mother of the kidneys. Its spirit name is *Truly Beautiful* (真美, Zhen Mei), and its official name is *Empty Completeness* (虚成, Xu Cheng). It is like a tiger and so expresses the Spirit. The lungs look like two suspended temple bells, and have the color white reflected by a red background. The lungs are located above the heart, opposite of the chest, and have six lobes.

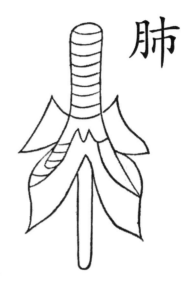

The Qi pulse of the lungs begins in the shoulder at *Central Mansion* (中府, Zhong Fu, Lu-1).

Comments

The lungs are located on either side of the chest (thorax), being a pair of sponge-like organs that fill with air. The trachea (windpipe), or as Chinese medicine refers to it, the Twelve Story Pagoda, leads the inhaled air into the lungs through tubular branches, called bronchi. During inhalation, the bronchi divide into smaller and smaller branches until becoming microscopic, ending in clusters called alveoli, from where the oxygen is absorbed into the blood. Carbon dioxide is a waste product of the metabolism. It travels with your blood back to the lungs and is diffused to the alveoli, where it is exhaled.

During inhalation the diaphragm (sitting beneath the lungs) is pushed downward, and returns upward during exhalation. If the diaphragm is injured or pinched, the lungs have great difficulty in functioning. For those who practice meditation, slouching of the chest can cause this, so it is important to maintain an upright position to allow the diaphragm to function freely.

White Tiger Kung

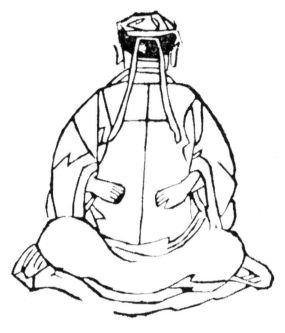

During autumn months the body is changing from a state of extreme Yang to Yin. The lungs are Yin organs and so are the first of all the organs to experience autumnal changes, being aggravated by the end of summer pollens in the air. This can cause the lungs to change from a state of Ultimate Yin to Young Yin. The lungs are associated with the Metal element. Metal produces Water, so taking in more fluids during this time is very beneficial to the lungs and helps them to maintain a proper state of Yin.

The kung to be performed in the three months of autumn [seventh, eighth, and ninth lunar months] are for nourishing and repairing the lungs.

[First sitting cross-legged and facing west] grasp the ground with both hands while contracting the body and bending forward. Then raise the body three times[48] to disperse the noxious Qi of the lungs and to repair old injuries that may have collected within them. Next, turn over the hands into fists and pound the back, left and right alternately. This will drive out trapped toxic air within the thorax. Pound the back at least 48 times or even 108 times. When done, close the eyes, knock the teeth [3x], and rise [to a standing position].

Face south, breathe in nine mouthfuls, and swallow nine times [嚥九息, Yan Jiu Xi].

If using Embryonic Breathing it will help lead the Qi from the internal organs out to the skin and so strengthen Protective Qi. Rub the chest several times, moving from the center to the outward sides of the chest, then massage the Lung Meridian.[49]

---

48 After bending forward and grasping the ground, return to the upright position. Repeat these bending forward and returning movements three times. Use Embryonic Breathing.

49 In the autumn and winter seasons, switch to massaging the right side of the body first, then the left. Remain standing when massaging the meridians in this kung.

Autumn

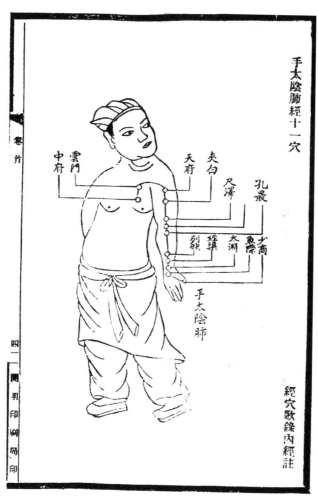

Ultimate Yin Hand Lung Meridian

Herbs for Cleansing and Nourishing the Lungs

Schisandra Fruit [五味子, Wu Wei Zi]

The Chinese name of this fruit translates as Five Flavors. Schisandra fruit (magnolia vine) beneficially supports the Lung Meridian and Kidney Meridian. High in antioxidants and helps prevent liver damage. The list of benefits for this fruit is quite extensive, but the reason it is recommended here is that it promotes saliva production, prevents coughing, enhances vascular relaxation, and reduces hypertension. It also corrects erectile dysfunction and spermatorrhea. Daily dosage: 1.5 to 3 grams.

Astragalus Root [黃耆, Huang Qi]

Proponents of astragalus claim it protects against heart disease. It is said to stimulate the spleen, liver, lungs, circulatory, and urinary systems. It is a natural dietary supplement used for treating the common cold, upper respiratory infections, fibromyalgia, diabetes, and to help improve overall weakness. It's also used to treat arthritis, asthma, and nervous conditions as well as to lower blood sugar and blood pressure. Daily dosage: 6 to 10 grams.

Asparagus Tuber [天門冬, Tian Men Dong]

The asparagus tuber is the underground portion of the asparagus plant. It enters the Lung and Kidney meridians. Its medical function is to arrest coughing, expel phlegm, and prevent bacteria in the lungs. It treats lungs experiencing dryness with no heat. Daily dosage: 10 to 20 grams.

Foods for Expelling Foul Airs (Detoxing) of the Lungs

Green Teas [綠茶, Lu Cha]

All green teas are high in antioxidants and so have a very cleansing effect on the lungs. High doses of green teas are not good for the lungs, so one or two cups of green tea per day is sufficient and beneficial.

Chinese Broccoli [芥蘭, Gai Lan]

Chinese broccoli is actually a leafy green vegetable, and is also considered as Chinese kale. Broccolini is actually a hybrid of gai lan and kale. Gai lan is harvested during the autumn and early winter season, and so best if eaten during these times. Like most leafy green vegetables, it is purifying for the lungs and liver. Gai lan has a very high content of antioxidants, more so than broccoli itself. It provides cardiovascular protection and contains many anti-cancer and anti-helicobacter compounds.

Carrots [胡蘿卜, Hu Luo Bo]

Carrots are abundant with vitamin A and beta-carotene, along with a variety of other vitamins and nutrients. Beta-carotene and lutein in carrots decrease the risk of heart disease and reduce cholesterol levels. Eating more carrots has shown to decrease the risk of stroke. Vitamin A in carrots, along with its antioxidants and beta-carotene slow down aging cells, improve eye sight, protect against sun damage, and prevent dryness of the skin, hair, and nails. Studies have shown that carrots are also helpful in fighting cancer of many types, and that smokers who ate carrots had a decreased risk of contracting lung cancer.

Six Dao Yin Seated Exercises for Autumn

First Autumn Exercise

立秋七月節

Establishing Summer—Seventh Moon

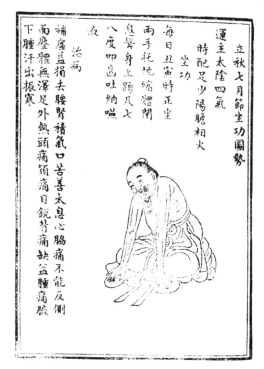

Dao Yin Exercise 13

Month: Seventh Moon
Days: 1st thru 14th
Hours: Chou (丑) 1:00 am to 3:00 am
Yin (寅) 3:00 am to 5:00 am.

坐 功
Seated Exercise

運主太陰四氣
Mobilize and control the Four Qi of Ultimate Yin.

Ultimate Yin is a reference to the organs and Qi of the lungs and spleen. *Mobilizing and controlling the Four Qi* of Ultimate Yin is then associated with both Metal and Earth, so within this exercise Metal and Earth stimulate the Four Qi—lungs and large intestine (Metal), and spleen and Triple Warmer (Earth).

時配足少陽膽相火
At this time enjoin the Young Yang Foot Meridian of the Gallbladder.

The meridian begins in the Qi point of *Moonlight Crevice* (瞳子髎, Tong Zi Liao, GB-1) and ends in *Yin Foot Cavity* (足竅陰, Zu Qiao Yin, GB-44).

On the right side of the body, rub the areas of these two points 36 times in a clockwise manner, starting with *Moonlight Crevice* and finishing with *Yin Foot Cavity*.

Autumn

Next, vigorously massage the pathway of the Young Yang Foot Meridian three times. Repeat on the left side of the body.

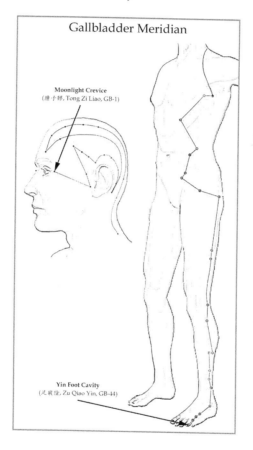

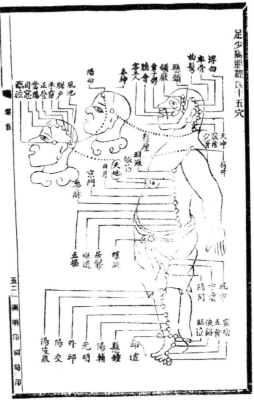

Young Yang Foot Meridian of the Gallbladder, 45 Qi Points[50]

相 火
Secondary Fire

At this time of year the Secondary Fire is too strong and must be regulated and brought into harmony. This is caused by insufficient Qi in the

---

50   Diagram indicates 45 Qi points, but modern texts list 44.

Young Yang Foot Gallbladder Meridian. The exercise is designed to help alleviate this problem.

If the heat of sexual desire becomes too strong, rub the middle of the soles of the feet, the *Bubbling Well* (湧泉, Yong Quan) Qi cavities, with the thumbs.

治病
Medicinal Cure

Remedies injured or weak parts of the body by filling them with Qi. Dispels bad airs collected in the loins and kidneys. Relieves pain in the heart and ribs, inability to turn the body easily, external heat of the feet, headaches, painful jaw, protrusion of the eyes, swollen and painful sternum and armpits, and cold perspiration.

旨示
Instructions

Seated, place both hands on the ground, contract the body, close the breath [閉氣, Bi Qi], and then raise the body in a jerking fashion. Repeat 56 times.

終功
Concluding Kung

Knock the Teeth [叩齒, Kou Chi] 36 times; perform 24 Blowing-Out and Drawing-In [吐納, Tu Na] breaths, and Swallow the Saliva [嚥液, Yan Ye] three times.

Second Autumn Exercise
處暑七月中
Ending Heat—Middle of Seventh Moon

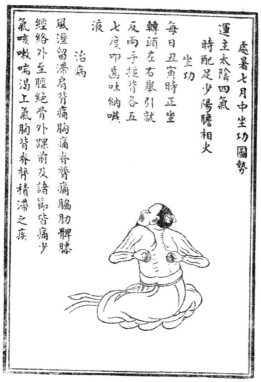

Dao Yin Exercise 14

Month: 7th Moon
Days: 15th thru 29th
Hours: Chou (丑) 1:00 to 3:00 am
Yin (寅) 3:00 to 5:00 am.

坐 功
Seated Exercise

運主太陰四氣
Mobilize and control the Four Qi of Ultimate Yin.

Ultimate Yin is a reference to the organs and Qi of the lungs and spleen. *Mobilizing and controlling the Four Qi* of Ultimate Yin is then associated with both Metal and Earth, so within this exercise Metal and Earth stimulate the Four Qi—lungs and large intestine (Metal), and spleen and Triple Warmer (Earth).

時配足少陽膽相火
At this time enjoin the Young Yang Foot Meridian of the Gallbladder.

The meridian begins in the Qi point of *Moonlight Crevice* (瞳子髎, Tong Zi Liao, GB-1) and ends in *Yin Foot Cavity* (足竅陰, Zu Qiao Yin, GB-44).

On the right side of the body, rub the areas of these two points 36 times in a clockwise manner, starting with *Moonlight Crevice* and finishing with *Yin Foot Cavity*.

Next, vigorously massage the pathway of the Young Yang Foot Meridian three times. Repeat on the left side of the body.

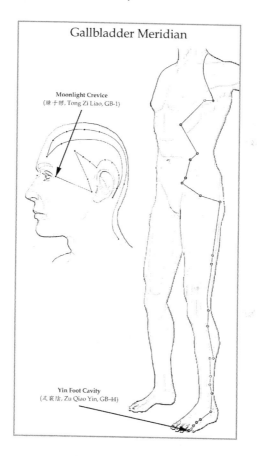

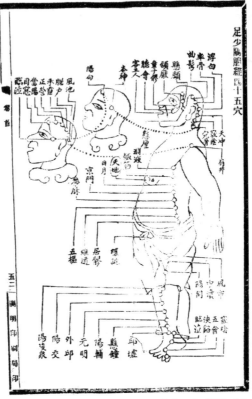

Young Yang Foot Meridian of the Gallbladder, 45 Qi Points[51]

相 火
Secondary Fire

At this time of year the Secondary Fire is too strong and must be regulated and brought into harmony. This is caused by insufficient Qi in the

---

51 Diagram indicates 45 Qi points, but modern texts list 44.

Young Yang Foot Gallbladder Meridian. The exercise is designed to help alleviate this problem.

If the heat of sexual desire becomes too strong, rub the middle of the soles of the feet, the *Bubbling Well* (湧泉, Yong Quan) Qi cavities, with the thumbs.

治病
Medicinal Cure
Remedies rheumatism and pain in the shoulders, back, chest, ribs, thighs, knees, and capillaries; pain on the outside legs and ankles; pain in the various joints; cough, asthma, shortness of breath, and thirst.

旨示
Instructions
Seated, raise the head and alternately turn it right and left while beating the back 35 times with the backs of both fists.

終功
Concluding Kung
Knock the Teeth [叩齒, Kou Chi] 36 times; perform 24 Blowing-Out and Drawing-In [吐納, Tu Na] breaths, and Swallow the Saliva [嚥液, Yan Ye] three times.

Third Autumn Exercise

白露八月節

White Dew—Eighth Moon

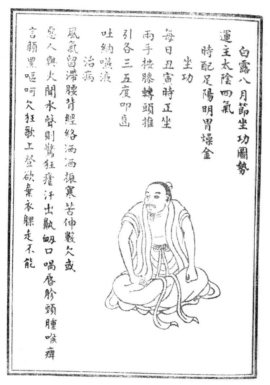

Dao Yin Exercise 15

Month: Eighth Moon
Days: 1st thru 14th
Hours: Chou (丑) 1:00 to 3:00 a.m.
Yin (寅) 3:00 to 5:00 a.m.

Chen Tuan's Four Season Internal Kungfu

坐功
Seated Exercise

運主太陰四氣
Mobilize and control the Four Qi of Ultimate Yin.

Ultimate Yin is a reference to the organs and Qi of the lungs and spleen. *Mobilizing and controlling the Four Qi* of Ultimate Yin is then associated with both Metal and Earth, so within this exercise Metal and Earth stimulate the Four Qi—lungs and large intestine (Metal), and spleen and Triple Warmer (Earth).

時配足陽明燥金
At this time enjoin the Bright Yang Foot Meridian.

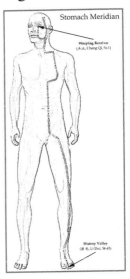

The meridian begins in the Qi point of *Weeping Receiver* (承泣, Cheng Qi, St-1) and ends in *History Valley* (歷兌, Li Dui, St-45).

On the right side of the body, rub the areas of these two points 36 times in a clockwise manner, starting with *Weeping Receiver* and finishing with *History Valley*.

Next, vigorously massage the pathway of the Bright Yang

Autumn

Foot Meridian three times. Repeat on the left side of the body.

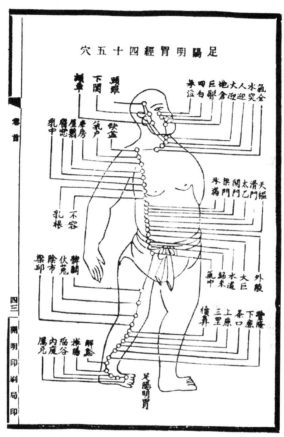

Bright Yang Foot Meridian of the Stomach, 45 Qi Points

燥金
Dry Metal

At this time of year the lungs (Metal) experience an excess of dryness because of insufficient Qi in the Bright Yang Foot Stomach Meridian. The exercise alleviates this problem.

Dryness in the lungs can also be exasperated from excessive seminal or menstrual dissipation.

治病
Medicinal Cure

Remedies rheumatism of the loins and back; lips turned dark in color; swelling in the neck; retching; mental disorders; and flushing of the face.

旨示
Instructions

Sit upright, press the two hands on the knees and push downward while turning the head, stretching it 15 times to each side [turning to the right first, then the left].

終功
Concluding Kung

Knock the Teeth [叩齒, Kou Chi] 36 times; perform 24 Blowing-Out and Drawing-In [吐納, Tu Na] breaths, and Swallow the Saliva [嚥液, Yan Ye] three times.

Fourth Autumn Exercise
秋分八月中

Autumn Equinox—Middle of Eighth Moon

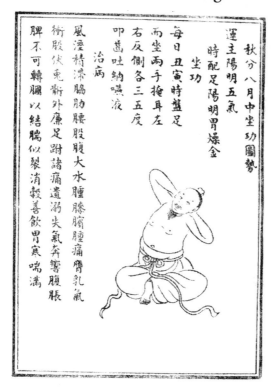

Dao Yin Exercise 16

Month: Eighth Moon
Days: 15th thru 30th
Hours: Chou (丑) 1:00 to 3:00 a.m.
Yin (寅) 3:00 to 5:00 a.m.

Chen Tuan's Four Season Internal Kungfu

坐功
Seated Exercise

運主陽明五氣
Mobilize and control the Five Qi of Bright Yang.

Bright Yang is a reference to the organs and Qi of the stomach and large intestine. *Mobilizing and controlling the Five Qi* of Bright Yang is then associated with both Earth and Metal, so within this exercise Earth and Metal stimulate the Five Qi —spleen, Triple Warmer, and stomach (Earth); large intestine and lungs (Metal).

時配足陽明燥金
At this time enjoin the Bright Yang Foot Meridian.

The meridian begins in the Qi point of *Weeping Receiver* (承泣, Cheng Qi, St-1) and ends in *History Valley* (歷兌, Li Dui, St-45).

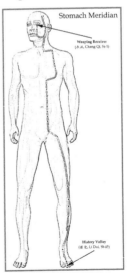

On the right side of the body, rub the areas of these two points 36 times in a clockwise manner, starting with *Weeping Receiver* and finishing with *History Valley*.

Next, vigorously massage the pathway of the Bright Yang

Foot Meridian three times. Repeat on the left side of the body.

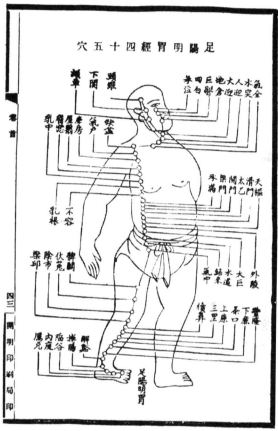

Bright Yang Foot Meridian of the Stomach, 45 Qi Points

燥金
Dry Metal

At this time of year the lungs (Metal) experience an excess of dryness because of insufficient Qi in the Bright Yang Foot Stomach Meridian. The exercise alleviates this problem.

Dryness in the lungs can also be exasperated from excessive seminal or menstrual dissipation.

治病
Medicinal Cure

Remedies rheumatism of the ribs, loins, thighs, and ankles; distention of the abdomen and rumbling of air; sensations of air colliding in the chest; pain in the thighs, legs, and ankles; incontinence of urine; stiffness in the thighs; very rapid digestion; coldness in the stomach; and great thirst.

旨示
Instructions

Sitting cross legged with both hands covering the ears, sway the body right and left 15 times to each side.

終功
Concluding Kung

Knock the Teeth [叩齒, Kou Chi] 36 times; perform 24 Blowing-Out and Drawing-In [吐納, Tu Na] breaths, and Swallow the Saliva [嚥液, Yan Ye] three times.

Fifth Autumn Exercise
寒露九月節
Cold Dew—Ninth Moon

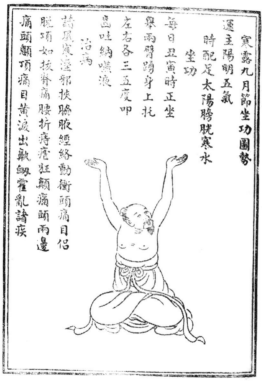

Dao Yin Exercise 17

Month: Ninth Moon
Days: 1st thru 14th
Hours: Chou (丑) 1:00 to 3:00 a.m.
Yin (寅) 3:00 to 5:00 a.m.

坐功
Seated Exercise

運主陽明五氣
Mobilize and control the Five Qi of Bright Yang.

Bright Yang is a reference to the organs and Qi of the stomach and large intestine. *Mobilizing and controlling the Five Qi* of Bright Yang is then associated with both Earth and Metal, so within this exercise Earth and Metal stimulate the Five Qi—spleen, Triple Warmer, and stomach (Earth); large intestine and lungs (Metal).

時配足太陽膀胱寒水
At this time enjoin the Ultimate Yang Foot Meridian of the Urinary Bladder.

The meridian begins in the Qi point of *Bright Eye* (睛明, Jing Ming, UB-1) and ends in *Foremost Yin* (至陰, Zhi Yin, UB-67).

On the right side of the body, rub the areas of these two points 36 times in a clockwise manner, starting with *Bright Eye* and finishing with *Foremost Yin*.

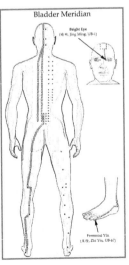

Next, vigorously massage the pathways of the Ultimate Yang Foot Meridian three times. Repeat on the left side of the body.

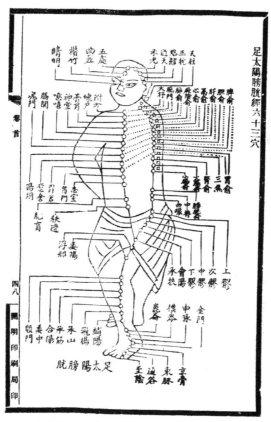

Ultimate Yang Foot Meridian of the Urinary Bladder, 63 Qi Points[52]

---

[52] Diagram indicates 63 Qi points, but modern texts list 67.

Cold Water

At this time of year the kidneys (Water) experience the excess of Cold Water because of coldness in the kidneys and insufficient Qi in the Ultimate Yang Foot Bladder Meridian. The exercise alleviates this problem.

治病
Medicinal Cure

Remedies bad winds; coldness and dampness; pain of the ribs, neck, loins, and spine; headaches; hemorrhoids, mental illness; and yellowness of the eyes.

旨示
Instructions

Sit upright, raise both hands over the head as if supporting something, then jerk the body left and right 35 times to each side.

終功
Concluding Kung

Knock the Teeth [叩齒, Kou Chi] 36 times; perform 24 Blowing-Out and Drawing-In [吐納, Tu Na] breaths, and Swallow the Saliva [嚥液, Yan Ye] three times.

Sixth Autumn Exercise

霜降九月中

Descending Frost—Middle of Ninth Moon

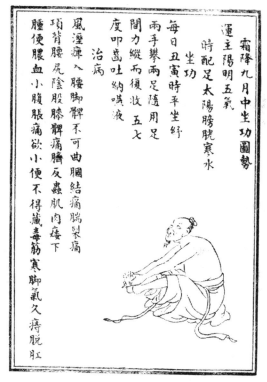

Dao Yin Exercise 18

Month: Ninth Moon
Days: 15th thru 30th
Hours: Chou (丑) 1:00 to 3:00 am
Yin (寅) 3:00 to 5:00 am

坐功
Seated Exercise

運主陽明五氣
Mobilize and control the Five Qi of Bright Yang.

Bright Yang is a reference to the organs and Qi of the stomach and large intestine. *Mobilizing and controlling the Five Qi* of Bright Yang is then associated with both Earth and Metal, so within this exercise Earth and Metal stimulate the Five Qi —spleen, Triple Warmer, and stomach (Earth); large intestine and lungs (Metal).

時配足太陽膀胱寒水
At this time enjoin the Ultimate Yang Foot Meridian of the Urinary Bladder.

The meridian begins in the Qi point of *Bright Eye* (睛明, Jing Ming, UB-1) and ends in *Foremost Yin* (至陰, Zhi Yin, UB-67).

On the right side of the body, rub the areas of these two points 36 times in a clockwise manner, starting with *Bright Eye* and finishing with *Foremost Yin*.

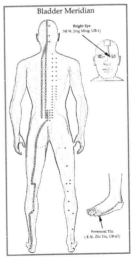

Next, vigorously massage the pathways of the Ultimate Yang Foot Meridian three times. Repeat on the left side of the body.

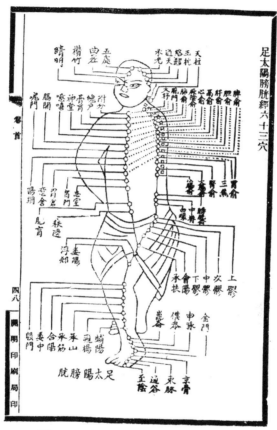

Ultimate Yang Foot Meridian of the Urinary Bladder, 63 Qi Points[53]

---

53 Diagram indicates 63 Qi points, but modern texts list 67.

寒水
Cold Water

At this time of year the kidneys (Water) experience the excess of Cold Water because of coldness in the kidneys and insufficient Qi in the Ultimate Yang Foot Bladder Meridian. The exercise alleviates this problem.

治病
Medicinal Cure

Remedies wind and dampness that enter into the loins; difficultly in extending and flexing the feet, thighs, and knees; muscular paralysis; a painful and distended abdomen; coldness in tendons; gout; hemorrhoids; and prolapsus ani.

旨示
Instructions

Sit evenly and stretch out the hands to seize the feet. Apply strength to the middle of the feet, then relax and draw back the hands [exhaling and lifting the feet off the ground]. Repeat 35 times.

終功
Concluding Kung

Knock the Teeth [叩齒, Kou Chi] 36 times; perform 24 Blowing-Out and Drawing-In [吐納, Tu Na] breaths, and Swallow the Saliva [嚥液, Yan Ye] three times.

Winter

Winter Kung
冬 功

Season of Storage for Repairing, Nourishing, and Strengthening the Kidneys

Black Tortoise
玄 龜

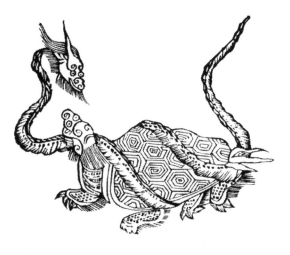

The celestial Black Tortoise represents the northern quadrant of the Heavens and the elemental activities of Water. The terrestrial representation of the kidneys is the image of a two-headed yellow deer.

Chen Tuan's Four Season Internal Kungfu

The Three Hexagrams Ruling the Winter Months

	#24	#19	#11	#34	#43	#1	#44	#33	#12	#20	#23	#2
	Fu	Lin	Tai	Da Zhuang	Guai	Qian	Gou	Dun	Pi	Guan	Bo	Kun
Earthly Branch	子 Zi	丑 Chou	寅 Yin	卯 Mao	辰 Chen	巳 Si	午 Wu	未 Wei	申 Shen	酉 You	戌 Xu	亥 Hai
Twelve Animals	Rat	Ox	Tiger	Rabbit	Dragon	Snake	Horse	Goat	Monkey	Rooster	Dog	Pig
Month	11	12	1	2	3	4	5	6	7	8	9	10
Hour	23-1	1-3	3-5	5-7	7-9	9-11	11-13	13-15	15-17	17-19	19-21	21-23

Tenth Moon	Eleventh Moon	Twelfth Moon
#2	#24	#19
Kun	Fu	Lin
Receptivity of Earth	*Returning*	*Approaching*

Animal Sign

Pig	Rat	Ox

Heavenly Stem

Hai (亥)	Zi (子)	Chou (丑)

Kidneys, 腎, Shen

The kidneys are the mother of the liver, and son of the lungs. The kidneys are situated opposite of and above the navel, residing in close contact with the lumbar spine.

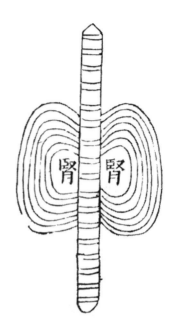

The name of the kidney spirit is *Water Spirit* (液神, Ye Shen) and both kidneys are designated as *Nourishing Infants* (養嬰, Yang Ying).

The mind-intent (意, Yi) is stored in the kidneys.

The kidneys are symbolized by a two-headed yellow deer, and resemble bean-shaped rounded stones. They are of the two colors of white silk reflected on purple.

The left kidney is the real one (origin of the regenerative forces in our bodies) and it interacts with the other Five Viscera. The right kidney is usually called the Gate of Life (命門, Ming Men). In males the right kidney is where the production of semen and sperm originate, and with females the fetal membrane and umbilical vesicle.

The Qi pulse of the kidneys begin in the middle of the soles of the feet, the *Bubbling Well* (湧泉, Yong Quan).

Comments

The kidneys are responsible for many functions of the human body, such as producing hormones, absorbing minerals, filtering the blood, and producing urine.

The kidneys govern the bones and marrow, and it is the marrow which when signaled by the kidneys will produce new red blood cells into the blood circulatory system.

Knocking the teeth and listening to the twenty-four breaths and the sound of swallowing the saliva are all methods that invigorate the kidneys.

The Bubbling Well points on the bottom of the feet regulate sexual desire. The sexual secretions (hormones) are connected to the kidneys. The kidneys do not actually contain semen or sperm, nor do they contain the fetal membrane or the umbilical vesicle. Rather, the sexual energy and pertinent hormones (of the endocrine system) derive from the kidneys. When they are dysfunctional or failing, sexual desire is quelled and sexual intercourse becomes impossible, as well as the production of semen and sperm, and the production of the fetal membrane or the umbilical vesicle. Hence, the reason the right kidney is called the Gate of Life, as no regeneration processes can occur without functional and healthy kidneys. However, if one kidney is removed or damaged, the other kidney will take on its functions.

Atop each kidney are the adrenal glands, which greatly influence and bring about the power needed for the Taoist practice of *Reverting Jing to Restore the Brain*.

Black Tortoise Kung

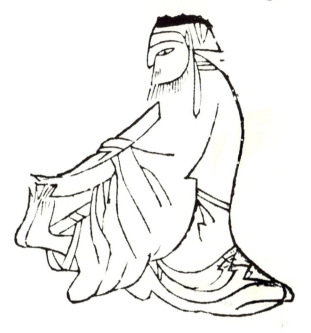

During winter months, the body is changing from a state of weak Yin to extreme Yin, and so a Qi deficiency occurs in the kidneys. The Protective Qi retreats to the center of the body causing the spirit to sink down from the heart making depression more apparent. The kidneys are associated with the Water element and so the Wood element [Jing] is very beneficial at this time.

For the winter months, sit [facing north] and grasp the toes of both feet with the hands 15 times. Next, rub the Bubbling Well points on the bottom of the feet 30 times.

Then, rub the kidneys with the back of the fists of both hands 30 times. Next, flick the back of the ear lobes 30 times. Place the thumbs along the neck, beneath the ears, and with the index and middle fingers, flick the ears while pressing the thumbs into the neck muscles on each side of the neck. This exercise strengthens the Ear Gates [耳門, Er Men].

Lastly, facing south, breathe in nine mouthfuls, and swallow nine times [嚥九息, Yan Jiu Xi].

The ears are the gateway for the Jing, and Jing is seated in the kidneys. Jing is dissipated through the ears, but when the hearing is turned inwards, the Jing is preserved, and thus the kidneys are repaired and nourished.

If using Embryonic Breathing allow the exhalation to be longer than the inhalation, causing the Protective Qi to increase and strengthen. Raise the spirit during this time and be more active physically.[54]

---

[54] Although it's not stated in Chen Tuan's text, massage the Kidney Meridian, starting on the right side first, then the left.

Winter

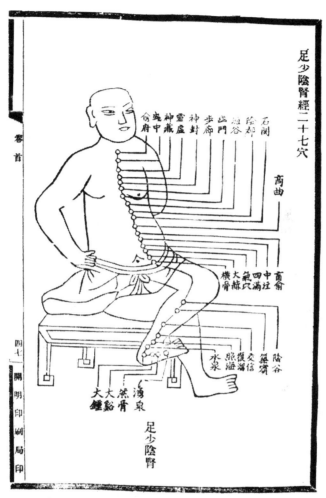

Young Yin Foot Meridian of the Kidneys

Herbs for Cleansing and Nourishing the Kidneys

Solomon's Seal [黃精, Huang Jing]

Enters Spleen, Lung, and Kidney meridians. Remedies weak digestion, lack of energy, tiredness, and dry cough, which can all be symptoms of winter months. Because of its effects on anti-stress, improvement of cardiac function, and its antibiotic function, Solomon's seal is considered in Taoism as a longevity herb. Daily dosage: 10 to 15 grams for decoction. Boil in water.

Licorice Root [甘草, Gan Cao]

Enters all twelve meridians. Tonifies the spleen, mobilizes the Qi, clears excessive heat, rids the body of toxins, expels phlegm and stops coughing, prevents joint and muscular pain, and works well with and enhances the effects of other herbs. Also, relieves the weakness from tiredness and lack of strength, remedies palpitations and shortness of breath, relieves cough with abundance of phlegm, and cures stomach and solar plexus pain. Because of its ability to rid the body of toxins, especially those of the liver and kidneys, this herb is recommended during the winter season. Plus it has a sweetness that promotes body warmth during winter months. Daily dosage: 9 to 12 grams.

Ginseng [人蔘, Ren Sen]

White American ginseng is best. Ginseng improves blood circulation to the heart and strengthens the immune system. Ginseng aids in the reduction of cholesterol and has shown positive effects on increasing the elasticity of blood vessels. Taoism considers it a longevity herb. Daily dosage: 30 to 50 grams.

Foods for Expelling Foul Airs (Detoxing) of the Kidneys

Parsley [歐芹, Ou Qin]

One of the major effects of parsley is its ability to improve bone health, thereby aiding in the support of cleansing the kidneys. Parsley is rich in vitamin K and it helps the body absorb calcium. But parsley must be eaten in moderation, as getting too much vitamin K can cause blood clotting. Overall, parsley has a high content of vitamins and nutrients that are very cleansing for the kidneys and liver.

Dandelion [蒲公英, Pu Gong Ying]

In the West, dandelion is often considered a weed, but the Chinese have long used it as a treatment for promoting urine production and decreasing swelling (inflammation), which aids in the support and purification of the kidneys. Dandelion is also used for treating numerous ailments such as gallstones, joint pain, eczema, and bruises. It serves as a laxative, skin toner, blood tonic, and generally as a digestive tonic. Roasted dandelion roots make an excellent coffee substitute.

Six Dao Yin Seated Exercises for Winter

First Winter Exercise

立冬十月節

Winter Begins—Tenth Moon

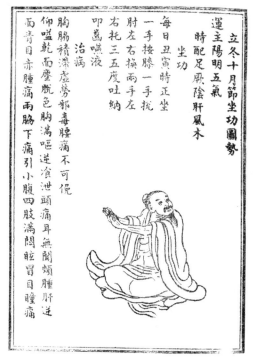

Dao Yin Exercise 19

Chen Tuan's Four Season Internal Kungfu

Month: Tenth Moon
Days: 1st thru 14th
Hours: Chou (丑) 1:00 to 3:00 a.m.
Yin (寅) 3:00 to 5:00 a.m.

坐功
Seated Exercise[55]

運主陽明五氣
Mobilize and control the Five Qi of Bright Yang.

Bright Yang is a reference to the organs and Qi of the stomach and large intestine. *Mobilizing and controlling the Five Qi* of Bright Yang is then associated with both Earth and Metal, so within this exercise Earth and Metal stimulate the Five Qi —spleen, Triple Warmer, and stomach (Earth); large intestine and lungs (Metal).

---

[55] This method is a combination of two other exercises: the first part is similar to Exercise 20, which stimulates the Faint Yin Foot Meridian of the Liver, and the second part is similar to Exercise 4, which stimulates the Bright Yang Hand Meridian of the Large Intestine. The liver and large intestine are the processors of the body, so the idea for performing these exercises at the beginning of the winter season is to aid the body in the processing and elimination of toxins. At this time of year, the body craves more grains, starches, sugars, and fats for warmth and for the storage of Jing (Essence).

Winter

時配足厥陰肝風木
At this time enjoin the Faint Yin Foot Meridian of the Liver.

The meridian begins in the Qi point of *Great Mound* (大敦, Da Dun, Lv-1) and ends in *Cyclic Door* (期門, Qi Men, Lv-14).

On the right side of the body, rub the areas of these two points 24 times in a clockwise manner, starting with *Great Mound* and finishing with *Cyclic Door*.

Next, vigorously massage the pathway of the Faint Yin Foot Meridian three times. Repeat on the left side of the body.

Chen Tuan's Four Season Internal Kungfu

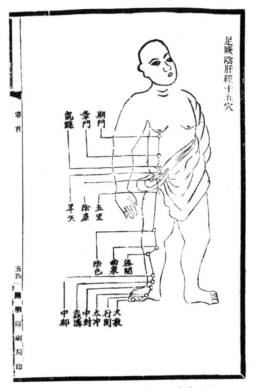

*Faint Yin Foot Meridian of the Liver,
15 Qi Points*[56]

風木
Wind Wood

At this time of year the liver (Wood) experiences an excess of Wind Wood because the Qi of the Faint Yin Foot Liver Meridian is insufficient. The exercise alleviates this problem.

---

56 Diagram indicates 15 Qi points, but modern texts list 14.

治病
Medicinal Cure

Remedies and relieves deficient saliva, nausea and hiccups, constipation, headaches, deafness, vertigo, and swollen jaws; red, swollen and painful eyes; feelings of depression affecting the abdomen, ribs, and the four extremities.

旨示
Instructions

Sit upright, place the right hand on the corresponding knee [pressing down slightly] with the other hand grasping the elbow [as though supporting it]. Alternate the hands right and left 15 times to each side.

Extend the right leg and position both arms to the left diagonal [holding them at chest level]. Turn the head right and left 42 times. Repeat to the other side, switching the leg and arm positions, and turning the head right and left 42 times.

終功
Concluding Kung

Knock the Teeth [叩齒, Kou Chi] 36 times; perform 24 Blowing-Out and Drawing-In [吐納, Tu Na] breaths, and Swallow the Saliva [嚥液, Yan Ye] three times.

Second Winter Exercise

小雪十月中

Lesser Snow—Middle of Tenth Moon

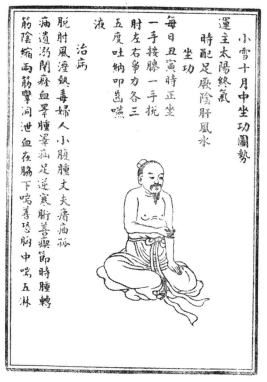

Dao Yin Exercise 20

Month: Tenth Moon
Days: 15th thru 29th
Hours: Chou (丑) 1:00 to 3:00 a.m.
Yin (寅) 3:00 to 5:00 a.m.

Chen Tuan's Four Season Internal Kungfu

坐功
Seated Exercise

運主太陽絡氣
Mobilize and control the Ultimate Yang blood and Qi channels.

Ultimate Yang represents the element of Fire and the production of heat within the entire body through what is called *Free Circulation of the Qi*. Ultimate Yang here not only refers to the Ultimate Yang Hand Meridian of the Small Intestine and the Ultimate Yang Foot Meridian of the Urinary Bladder, but to the other ten meridians of the body and the entire blood circulatory system as well.

時配足厥風木
At this time enjoin the Faint Yin Foot Meridian of the Liver.

The meridian begins in the Qi point of *Great Mound* (大敦, Da Dun, Lv-1) and ends in *Cyclic Door* (期門, Qi Men, Lv-14).

On the right side of the body, rub the areas of these two points 24 times in a clockwise manner, starting with *Great Mound* and finishing with *Cyclic Door*.

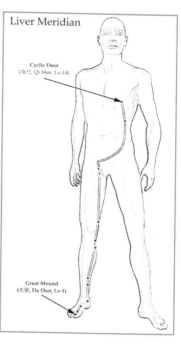

Next, vigorously massage the pathway of the Faint Yin Foot Meridian three times. Repeat on the left side of the body.

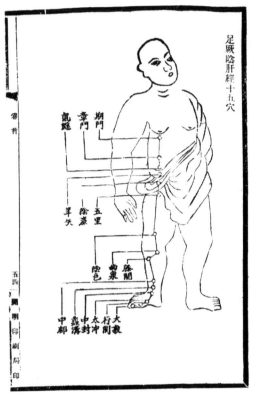

Faint Yin Foot Meridian of the Liver, 15 Qi Points[57]

風木
Wind Wood

At this time of year the liver (Wood) experiences an excess of Wind Wood because the Qi of the Faint Yin Foot Liver Meridian is insufficient. The exercise alleviates this problem.

---

57 Diagram indicates 15 Qi points, but modern texts list 14.

治病
Medicinal Cure
Remedies enlargement of the female's small abdomen and hernias in males; incontinence of urine; swelling of joints; contracted tendons; small membrum virile; gonorrhea of the mouth, penis or vagina, cervix, throat, and eyes; fullness in the chest; fright; and asthma affecting the lower ribs.

旨示
Instructions
Sit upright, place the right hand on the corresponding knee [pressing down slightly] with the other hand grasping the elbow [as though supporting it]. Alternate the hands right and left 15 times to each side.

終功
Concluding Kung
Knock the Teeth [叩齒, Kou Chi] 36 times; perform 24 Blowing-Out and Drawing-In [吐納, Tu Na] breaths, and Swallow the Saliva [嚥液, Yan Ye] three times.

Third Winter Exercise

大雪十一月節

Great Snow—Eleventh Moon

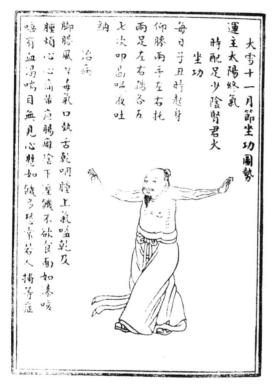

Dao Yin Exercise 21

Month: Eleventh Moon
Days: 1st thru 14th
Hours: Zi (子) 11:00 p.m. to 1:00 a.m.
Chou (丑) 1:00 to 3:00 a.m.

坐 功
Seated Exercise[58]

運主太陽絡氣
Mobilize and control the Ultimate Yang blood and Qi channels.

Ultimate Yang represents the element of Fire and the production of heat within the entire body through what is called *Free Circulation of the Qi*. Ultimate Yang here not only refers to the Ultimate Yang Hand Meridian of the Small Intestine and the Ultimate Yang Foot Meridian of the Urinary Bladder, but to the other ten meridians of the body and the entire blood circulatory system as well.

---

[58] Even though the text indicates the exercise is seated, the instructions call to stand for this one.

Winter

時配足少陰腎君火
At this time enjoin the Young Yin Foot Meridian of the Kidneys.

The meridian begins in the Qi point of *Bubbling Well* (湧泉, Yong Quan, K-1) and ends in *Shu Mansion* (俞府, Shu Fu, K-27).

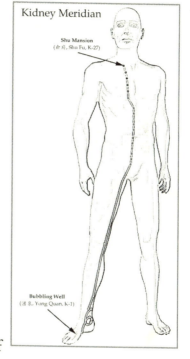

On the right side of the body, rub the areas of these two points 24 times in a clockwise manner, starting with the *Bubbling Well* and finishing with *Shu Mansion*.

Next, vigorously massage the pathway of the Young Yin Foot Meridian three times. Repeat on the left side of the body.

Chen Tuan's Four Season Internal Kungfu

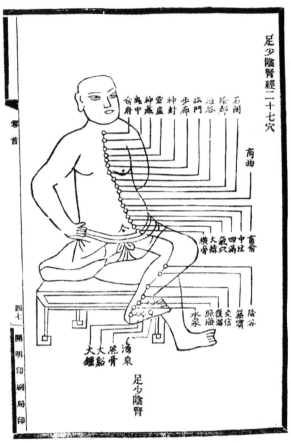

Young Yin Foot Meridian of the Kidneys,
27 Qi Points

Winter

君火
Ruling Fire

At this time of year the heart (Fire) experiences an excess of Fire because the Qi of the Young Yin Foot Kidney Meridian is insufficient. The exercise alleviates this problem.

治病
Medicinal Cure

Remedies wind and dampness of the feet and knees; heat in the mouth and dryness of the tongue; swelling of the throat; jaundice; hunger without appetite; cough; asthma; and fright.

旨示
Instructions

Stand upright with the knees locked. Both hands are extended out to the sides as though supporting the two feet [for balance]. Then stamp the feet right and left each 35 times.

終功
Concluding Kung

Knock the Teeth [叩齒, Kou Chi] 36 times; perform 24 Blowing-Out and Drawing-In [吐納, Tu Na] breaths, and Swallow the Saliva [嚥液, Yan Ye] three times.

Fourth Winter Exercise

冬至十一月中

Winter Solstice—Middle of Eleventh Moon

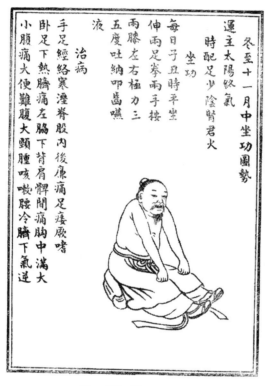

Dao Yin Exercise 22

Month: Eleventh Moon
Days: 15th thru 30th
Hours: Zi (子) 11:00 p.m. to 1:00 a.m.
Chou (丑) 1:00 to 3:00 a.m.

Chen Tuan's Four Season Internal Kungfu

坐功
Seated Exercise

運主太陽終氣
Mobilize and control the Ultimate Yang blood and Qi channels.

Ultimate Yang represents the element of Fire and the production of heat within the entire body through what is called *Free Circulation of the Qi*. Ultimate Yang here not only refers to the Ultimate Yang Hand Meridian of the Small Intestine and the Ultimate Yang Foot Meridian of the Urinary Bladder, but to the other ten meridians of the body and the entire blood circulatory system as well.

Winter

時配足少陰腎君火
At this time enjoin the Young Yin Foot Meridian of the Kidneys.

The meridian begins in the Qi point of *Bubbling Well* (湧泉, Yong Quan, K-1) and ends in *Shu Mansion* (俞府, Shu Fu, K-27).

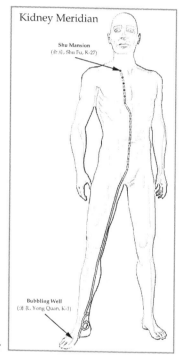

On the right side of the body, rub the areas of these two points 24 times in a clockwise manner, starting with the *Bubbling Well* and finishing with *Shu Mansion*.

Next, vigorously massage the pathway of the Young Yin Foot Meridian three times. Repeat on the left side of the body.

Chen Tuan's Four Season Internal Kungfu

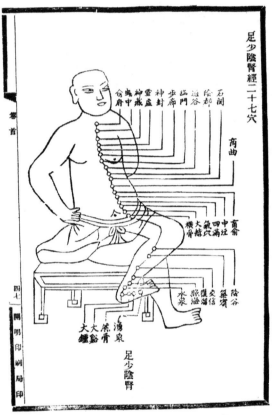

Young Yin Foot Meridian of the Kidneys, 27 Qi Points

君火
Ruling Fire

At this time of year the heart (Fire) experiences an excess of Fire because the Qi of the Young Yin Foot Kidney Meridian is insufficient. The exercise alleviates this problem.

治病
Medicinal Cure

Remedies cold dampness in the hands, feet, spine and thighs; pain within the lower ribs, between the shoulders, and middle of the thighs; swelling in the throat; distention of the abdomen; cough; loins that feel like cold water and are swollen; the breath below the navel that does not feel harmonious; acute pain beneath the navel; diarrhea; swollen feet; and dysentery.

旨示
Instructions

Sit evenly and extend both feet forward. Grasp the hands firmly, then press down on the area above the kneecaps, doing so with strength 15 times.

終功
Concluding Kung

Knock the Teeth [叩齒, Kou Chi] 36 times; perform 24 Blowing-Out and Drawing-In [吐納, Tu Na] breaths, and Swallow the Saliva [嚥液, Yan Ye] three times.

Fifth Winter Exercise

小寒十二月節

Lesser Cold—Twelfth Moon

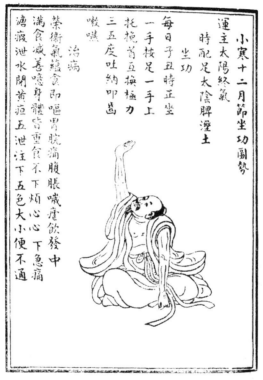

Dao Yin Exercise 23

Month: Twelfth Moon
Days: 1st thru 14th
Hours: Zi (子) 11:00 p.m. to 1:00 a.m.
Chou (丑) 1:00 to 3:00 a.m.

Chen Tuan's Four Season Internal Kungfu

坐功
Seated Exercise

運主太陽終氣
Mobilize and control the Ultimate Yang blood and Qi channels.

Ultimate Yang represents the element of Fire and the production of heat within the entire body through what is called *Free Circulation of the Qi*. Ultimate Yang here not only refers to the Ultimate Yang Hand Meridian of the Small Intestine and the Ultimate Yang Foot Meridian of the Urinary Bladder, but to the other ten meridians of the body and the entire blood circulatory system as well.

時配足太陰脾渴土
At this time enjoin the Ultimate Yin Foot Meridian of the Spleen.

The meridian begins in the Qi point of *Hidden White* (隱白, Yin Bai, Sp-1) and ends in *Great Control* (大包, Da Bao, Sp-21).

On the right side of the body, rub the areas of these two points in clockwise directions 24 times, starting with *Hidden White* and finishing with *Great Control*.

Next, vigorously massage the pathway of the Ultimate Yin Foot Meridian three times. Repeat on the left side of the body.

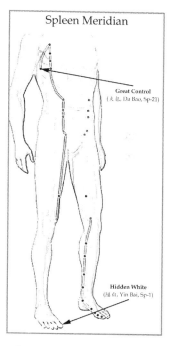

Chen Tuan's Four Season Internal Kungfu

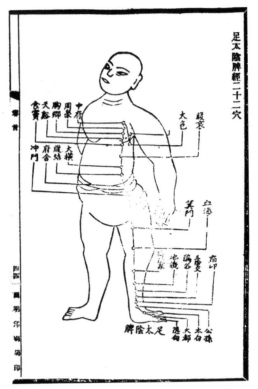

Ultimate Yin Foot Meridian of the Spleen, 22 Qi Points[59]

渴土
Parched Earth

At this time of year the Triple Warmer (Earth) experiences excess aridness because the Qi of the Ultimate Yin Foot Spleen Meridian is insufficient. The exercise alleviates this problem.

---

59 Diagram indicates 22 Qi points, but modern texts list 21.

治病
Medicinal Cure

Remedies air in the arteries and veins; vomiting; stomach ache; distended abdomen; swelling of the throat; decreased appetite; sighing; heaviness of the body; grief; diarrhea; obstructed urination; jaundice; five types and colors of diarrhea; dry mouth; indolence; excessive lying down; and lack of appetite.

旨示
Instructions

Sit upright with the left hand pressing on the right foot and the right hand raised over the head as if supporting something. Turn the head to look at the raised hand. Use strength in pressing and supporting while alternately turning the head and changing the hands 15 times to each side.

終功
Concluding Kung

Knock the Teeth [叩齒, Kou Chi] 36 times; perform 24 Blowing-Out and Drawing-In [吐納, Tu Na] breaths, and Swallow the Saliva [嚥液, Yan Ye] three times.

Sixth Winter Exercise

大寒十二月中

Great Cold—Middle of Twelfth Moon

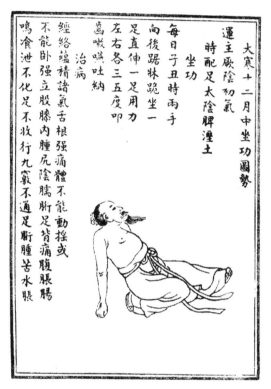

Dao Yin Exercise 24

Month: Twelfth Moon
Days: 15th thru 30th
Hours: Zi (子) 11:00 p.m. to 1:00 a.m.
Chou (丑) 1:00 to 3:00 a.m.

Chen Tuan's Four Season Internal Kungfu

坐功
Seated Exercise

運主厥陰初氣
Mobilize and control the Faint Yin to initiate New Qi.

Faint Yin is referencing the organs and Qi of the liver and pericardium. Through the exercise, *New Yang Qi* is being stimulated to control the effects of the old Faint Yin Qi acquired during the winter months. Faint Yin Qi is controlled in the last period of the year through initiating Ultimate Yin Qi and stimulating the Qi of the spleen.

時配足太陰脾渴土
At this time enjoin the Ultimate Yin Foot Meridian of the Spleen.

The meridian begins in the Qi point of *Hidden White* (隱白, Yin Bai, Sp-1) and ends in *Great Control* (大包, Da Bao, Sp-21).

On the right side of the body, rub the areas of these two points in clockwise directions 24 times, starting with *Hidden White* and finishing with *Great Control*.

Next, vigorously massage the

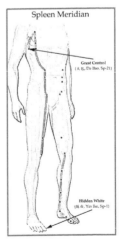

pathway of the Ultimate Yin Foot Meridian three times. Repeat on the left side of the body.

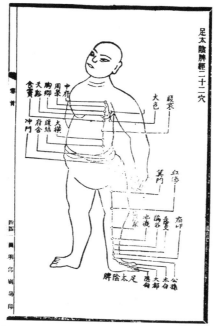

Ultimate Yin Foot Meridian of the Spleen, 22 Qi Points[60]

渴土
Parched Earth

At this time of year the Triple Warmer (Earth) experiences excess aridness because the Qi of the Ultimate Yin Foot Spleen Meridian is insufficient. The exercise alleviates this problem.

---

60   Diagram indicates 22 Qi points, but modern texts list 21.

治病
Medicinal Cure
Remedies and clears obstructions in all the capillaries; hardness, pain, or immobility in the root of the tongue; difficulty in moving or lying down; difficulty in exerting strength; swollen thighs; painful pelvis, thighs, legs, feet, and spine; distention of the abdomen; rumbling in the intestines; undigested food causing diarrhea; difficulty in moving the feet for walking; fluids unable to pass through the nine apertures.

旨示
Instructions
Both hands are placed behind the body with the right foot extended forward and the left foot folded underneath the body. With strength, stretch the right foot out while leaning back and looking upwards. Perform 15 times with the right foot, then repeat with the left foot [folding the right foot underneath the body].

終功
Concluding Kung
Knock the Teeth [叩齒, Kou Chi] 36 times; perform 24 Blowing-Out and Drawing-In [吐納, Tu Na] breaths, and Swallow the Saliva [嚥液, Yan Ye] three times.

Taoist Supine Methods

Chen Tuan
Two Supine Methods
陳摶睡法

The Taoist supine methods in this section come from the *The Book of Immortal Longevity of Ten Thousand Years.* The first two are attributed to Chen Tuan, while the others seem to be variants on his methods, with one practice exclusively for women and another exclusively for men. Supine methods are really useful, especially for healing sexual dysfunctions and restoring sexual energy (Jing) in the body.

The meditation method can initially be problematic since the body associates lying down with sleep, and therefore it can take added effort to keep the mind focusing on the breath. With practice, however, this can become a very profound and effective manner for meditation.

Lying on the Right Side Kung
右睡功圖

There are two methods for the *Lying on the Right Side Kung*.⁶¹ One is for restoring Jing (sexual energy) and the other is the supine meditation. The herbal formula *Divine Powder* (靈沙, Ling Sha), not shown here, is also associated with this kung. It produces perspiration and strengthens the heart.

Usually, the cultivator will perform the *Restoring the Jing* method once and then change the hands and feet to perform the Supine Meditation.

Restoring the Jing Method

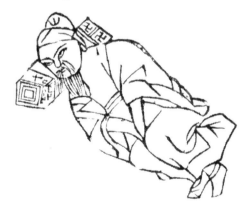

---

61   Also called *Chen Tuan Attaining the Great Sleep Kung* (陳摶得大睡功).

Lying on the right side of the body, bring up both knees as if in a fetal position and cross the left ankle over the right. Prop the head on a pillow to prevent strain in the neck.

Rub the palms together until warm, then place them so they embrace the penis and groin [membrum virile and scrotum]. In this position, circulate the Qi in the mouth 24 times [運氣口, Yun Qi Kou],[62] and then gently imagine the Qi descending into the lower Elixir Field. Repeat if desired, but warm the hands before beginning another 24 breaths.

Supine Meditation Method
Lying upon the right side of the body, flex the right leg and bend it back slightly. Extend the left leg, also slightly bending it and rest it over the right knee. The left hand rests upon the left thigh, and the right-hand palm is placed over the right ear (like cupping the ear). The head should be propped up on a pillow to prevent strain in the neck. Using Embryonic Breathing, focus on the lower Elixir Field.[63]

---

62 See *Preliminary Instructions* p. 78.

63 The illustration shows Chen Tuan visualizing or having an immortal visitation by the Jade Maiden during supine meditation. The Jade Maiden (玉女, Yu Nu) is the protector of immortals, and in Taoist lore she appears to those who have just achieved immortality.

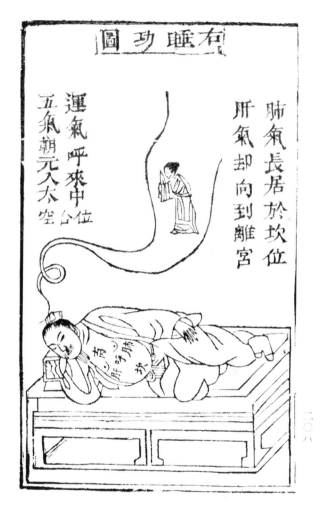

Illustration Translation

The Qi of the lungs dwells in the position of Kan.
肺氣長居於坎位

The lungs represent the Metal element, and Metal produces Water. The trigram for Water (☵, *Kan*) has one Yang line in its center and two Yin lines surrounding it, showing Heaven (☰, *Qian*) within the Earth (☷, *Kun*). Water (☵) symbolizes the Moon, which controls the ocean tides of the Earth. The lungs represent the autumn season and are classified as a Yin organ.

The liver Qi is directed to the Palace of Li.
肝氣却向到離宮

The liver represents the element of Wood and Wood produces Fire. The trigram for Fire (☲, *Li*) has one Yin line in its center and two Yang lines surrounding it, showing Earth (☷) within Heaven (☰). Fire (☲) symbolizes the sun, which gives warmth to Earth and brings light to the Heavens (sky). The liver represents the spring season and is classified as a Yang organ.

These two verses are pointing out several important correlations and ideologies: First is the elemental activity of Metal creating Water, Water creating Wood, and Wood creating Fire. Second, they convey the interdependence of the lungs and liver, of their being the father (liver) and mother (lungs), their trigram correlations to the sun (☲) and moon (☵), and of True Mercury (Metal Element) and True Lead (Water Element). Third, the lungs are home to the Earthly Spirit (魄, Po, also called the *White Spirit* and *Yin Spirit*), and the

Taoist Supine Methods

liver houses the Heavenly Spirit (魂, Hun, also called the *Cloud Spirit* and *Yang Spirit*).[64] Fourth, the lungs in Internal Alchemy represent the "bellows" (directed air) and the liver the "fuel" (the firewood).

The gist of these first two verses is to convey the physical and spiritual dualistic concepts of Yin and Yang within the body, and the next two verses relate the sublimation of these dual forces into one place (the Elixir Field), bringing all Five Qi together to enter the Tao. The Five Qi are the spiritual energies, or as they are called in Internal Alchemy "the reverted forces" of Essence (精, Jing), Spirit (神, Shen), Heavenly Spirit (魂, Hun), Earthly Spirit (魄, Po), and Mind-Intent (意, Yi). On the body, the Five Qi represent the liver, exhalation, lungs, Brightness/Fire (☲), and Abyss/Water (☵).

Mobilize the Qi, so when exhaling they arrive in the center, joining together in this position.
運氣呼來中合位

The center is the Elixir Field. The text points out that it is during exhalation when the Qi of the

---

[64] See *Actions & Retributions: A Taoist Treatise on Attaining Spiritual Virtue, Longevity, and Immortality* (Valley Spirit Arts, 2015) for a fuller explanation of the Hun and Po spirits.

lungs and liver (Kan ☵ and Li ☲) unite in the Elixir Field, or more simply, the exhalation is like a bellows blowing air onto the burning coals of the firewood to create a stronger fire to heat the furnace, thereby heating the mixture within the cauldron. Or, in this case, bringing all Five Qi together as one.

From the original court of the Five Qi, enter the Supreme Void.
五氣朝元入太空

> The *original court* is in the head, from the center of the brain into the Bai Hui (百回) cavern, the fontanel area. It is from here where the spirit can enter the Supreme Void.

Chen Xiyi's Lying on the Left Side Kung
陳希夷左睡功圖

This kung[65] is for the cure of excessive and involuntary ejaculation (spermatorrhea), a symptom of a kidney Qi problem. An herbal formula, *Spirit Herbal Soup* (神芎, Shen Xiong), not shown here, is also associated with this method.

The Method

Lie on the left side of the body, and when feeling a pending emission or excessive desire to ejaculate, bring the left middle finger to plug the right nostril. Then bring the right-hand middle finger to press upon the Tail Passageway [尾路, Wei Lu] cavity [tailbone], this is where the seminal vessel is located. In this position, circulate the Qi with six mouthfuls.[66] This will prevent the flow of semen.

---

[65] Also called, *Chen Xiyi's The Body of a Fallen Ox Gazing at the Moon* (陳希夷降牛望月形). Chen Xiyi is a stylized name of Chen Tuan.

[66] This is the practice of Yun Qi Kou (see p. 78) with the addition of gathering the Qi in the mouth first before circulating it. To breathe in *six mouthfuls* means visualizing the breath/Qi as being a white cloudy substance filling the mouth as you inhale and exhale six times. You aren't ingesting or circulating the Qi yet, but "gathering" it to fill the mouth. After six cycles of gathering it, you then circulate it six times with the Yun Qi Kou method.

Chen Tuan's Four Season Internal Kungfu

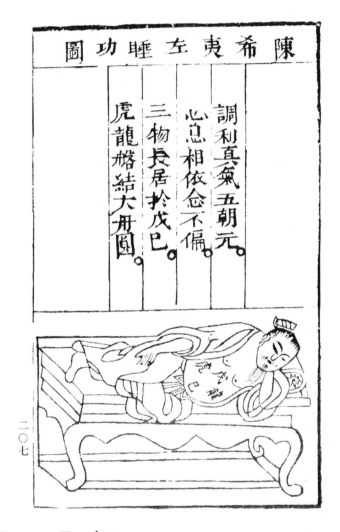

Illustration Translation

Harmonize the origin of the Five Courts to benefit from True Qi.

調利真氣五朝元

The *origin of the Five Courts* is a reference to the Five Viscera. When harmonized, they bring forth the True Qi.

The mind and breath are interdependent. Do not deviate from this thought.
心息相依念不偏

The mind leads the breath, and the mind functions because of the breath. *Do not deviate from this thought* means to keep this principle in mind. Some cultivators tend to think everything is in the mind, and so forget the importance of breath, and some just focus on the breath and forget that the mind is what leads the breathing.

The Three Things constantly reside in Wu and Ji.
三物長居於戊己

The *Three Things* are body, breath, and mind—Essence, Vitality, and Spirit. These are forever part of and dwell in *Wu and Ji,* the center (or the Earth) of a person.

The Tiger and Dragon move back and forth creating a strong sturdy vessel.
虎龍般結大舟固

This is to say, the Yin and Yang interplay with each other. When one reaches fullness it reverts to the other—Yin becomes Yang, and Yang becomes Yin.

From mobilizing the Qi *(moving back and forth)* the body becomes like a *strong and sturdy vessel* from which a person can transverse through the stages of Internal Alchemy to become immortal. On the body, *Wu* (戊) is the upper center. *Ji* (己) is the lower center. *Dragon* (龍) is the left side (Yang), and *Tiger* (虎) is the right.

Other Supine Methods

Taoist Priestess Huang Hua's Sleeping on Ice Pose
黃花姑睡冰圖

[Exclusively for Females]

For the cure of consumption and for lessening excess sexual desire causing extreme physical weakness and for the reduction of the menstrual flow. Herbal formula (not shown) is *Great Shop Soup* (大店湯, Da Dian Tang), which is meant for strengthening the thorax and strengthening the female reproduction system.

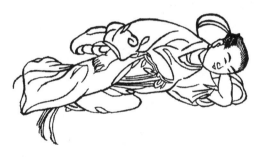

The Method

Lie upon your left side and use the left arm like a pillow. Rub the abdomen vigorously with the right fist. Push out the breasts and contract the abdomen when inhaling.[67] Relax the breasts and expand the abdomen when exhaling. Extend the right foot and leg slightly, pressing

---

67 Use *Embryonic Breathing* (胎息, Tai Xi) with this method.

it a little into the left leg, as though in a sleeping posture. Breathe in 32 mouthfuls of Qi, and then circulate the Qi in the mouth 12 times.⁶⁸

Yin Qinghe's Sleeping Method
尹清和睡法

Cures weaknesses in the spleen and stomach, and helps with indigestion. Herbal formula (not shown) is *Strengthening Spleen Pills* (壯脾丸, Zhuang Pi Wan).

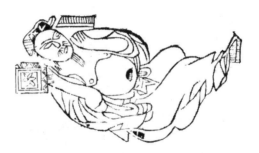

The Method
Lie on the back, resting the right foot across the left. Place both hands directly upon the shoulders and use Embryonic Breathing to expand and contract the abdomen. Circulate the Qi with six mouthfuls.

---

68   See note 66, but this time you are Embryonically Breathing 32 mouthfuls of Qi before circulating it 12 times with Yun Qi Kou.

Taoist Supine Methods

Celestial Master Xu Jing's Sleeping Kung
虛靜天師睡功

[Exclusively for Males]

This exercise is sometimes attributed to Chen Tuan, and simply called either *The Sleeping Method* (睡法, Shui Fa) or *The Sleeping Exercise of Chen Tuan* (陳摶睡功, Chen Tuan Shui Kung)—but the original text credits the exercise to Master Xu Jing.[69] It's used for the cure of nocturnal emissions. Herbal formula (not shown) is called *Nourishing the Heart Soup* (養心湯, Yang Xin Tang).

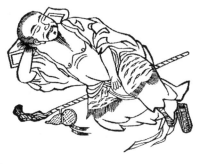

The Method

Recline obliquely on a high pillow, with the right hand placed underneath the head for support. Draw up the legs, with the right leg higher than the left. Press the left leg a little into the right leg. Use gentle Embryonic Breathing, empty the mind of extraneous thoughts,

---

[69] Master Xu Jing was a teacher of Li Qingyun. See *The Immortal: True Accounts of the 250-Year-Old Man, Li Qingyun* by Yang Sen (Valley Spirit Arts, 2014).

and breathe in 32 mouthfuls of Qi into the abdomen, doing so twelve times.⁷⁰

There are three variants of this exercise (not shown).

Chen's Natural Attainment of the Great Sleeping Kung
陳自得大睡功

This method is used to cure the excess of Cold Water, which occurs seasonally four times a year.⁷¹

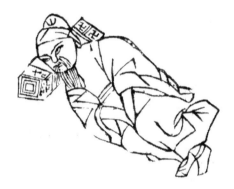

---

70 This means you are visualizing and breathing in mouthfuls of Qi as in the other exercises, but 12 sets of 32 mouthfuls. In other words, you are gathering the Qi in 384 breaths. This is just the idea of breathing in the white cloudy Qi, but not ingesting or circulating it.

71 The excess of *Cold Water* occurs four times in the year: during the final months of spring and autumn (third and ninth lunar months), spanning the seasons of *Bright Purity, Corn Rain, Cold Dew,* and *Descending Frost*. See Dao Yin Exercises 5, 6, 17, and 18.

The Method

Recline on the right side of the body, bringing up both legs by bending the knees upwards towards the stomach. The left ankle hooks around the right ankle. Rub the hands until hot, and then embrace the penis and groin [or place the hands over the vagina]. Mobilize the Qi to produce 24 mouthfuls.[72]

---

[72] Because the instruction says "*Mobilize the Qi,*" *this means* to first gather 24 mouthfuls of Qi and then circulate it 24 times.

Medicinal Kung Regimes

The two Medicinal Kung in this section are found in *The Book of Immortal Longevity of Ten Thousand Years* and other related works. In the forty-eight traditional Medicinal Kung documents, each contains an exercise, herbal formula, and related poetic verses.

The Medicinal Kung are a collection of exercises coming from various Taoist adepts of antiquity. When time permits, more of these works will be published on the Sanctuary of Tao website and eventually published in a future book. Here are the two methods most important to those who practice meditation on a regular basis.

Please be advised not to attempt to concoct the herbal formulas. If you wish to make use of them, please consult a Chinese herbalist and have them prepare it for you, also letting them know of any medications you are on. These formulas are very powerful and if used incorrectly can cause harm.

If you have any medical condition, please consult your physician prior to undertaking these Medicinal Kung regimes.

The Venerable Sovereign Li Playing the Lute Pose
李老君撫琴圖

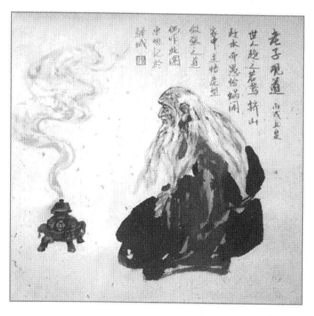

Lao Zi (Li Lao Jun)

Li Lao Jun (李老君) is Lao Zi (老子), or in many Taoist texts just Lao Jun (老君, Venerable Sovereign), the attributed founder of Taoism and author of the *Scripture on Tao and Virtue* (道德經, *Tao De Jing*). The surname Li (李) is thought to be his older former sobriquet, from the tale that he was born under a plum tree (李樹, Li Shu).

Cures
Chronic illnesses [从病, Zong Bing] and Yellow Swelling [黃腫, Huang Zhong].

Exercise
Sit silently with both hands pressed into the knees, and then rubbing them with vigor. Keep to the imagination for processing the Qi to all parts of the body. Then Mobilize Qi in 49 mouthfuls.[73] The Qi will then penetrate the blood and harmonize it, and the illness will then vanish.

Aside from this exercise being a cure for the mentioned illnesses, it is also very good for those meditators who experience pain in the legs from sitting. This is a very good exercise for stimulating the blood and Qi.

Herbal Formula
Iron Date Pills (棗礬丸, Zao Fan Wan)
Ingredients: 綠礬, Lu Fan (煅過, Duan Guo, burnt); 皮, Chen Pi (三錢, San Qian, 3 mace); 蒼朮, Cang Shu (各二兩, Ge Er Liang, each 2 ounces); 砂仁, Sha Ren (三錢, San Qian, 3 mace); 乾姜, Qian Jiang (dried ginger); 枳殼, Zhi Ke (三錢, San Qian, 3 mace); 檳榔, Bin Lang

---

[73] See note 72, p. 281.

(三錢, San Qian, 3 mace); and 人參, Ren Shen (三錢, San Qian, 3 mace).

Preparation
First boil the red dates,[74] then beat them so they become pulp. Powder all the other ingredients and mix them into the red-date paste. Fashion into pills. Take 49 pills in the morning and 49 in the evening mixed within rice gruel. Do not add fish, fowl, cold and raw articles, or anything with fat, as these will diminish the effects of the pills.

The Verses Say (詩曰, *Shi Yue*)

The Supreme Ultimate is not yet divided, transport the Yin.
太極未分運是陰

> The *Supreme Ultimate* is the Yin and Yang in their fixed positions and so are undivided. They separate when the Yin is mobilized. The Yang cannot be moved unless the Yin is mobilized. This is expressing Lao Zi's idea of *Wei Wu Wei*, action

---

[74] There was an error in the original Chinese text concerning the first character of the formula name. The text had *Dong* (東), meaning the East, but the actual character is supposed to be *Zao* (棗), meaning "dates," Chinese red dates, or more commonly called, jujube. The second character was also written incorrectly. The character da (大) in the middle of the ideogram was missing. As it was written, there was no such ideogram in Chinese. These types of errors occur somewhat frequently in older handwritten texts.

through non-action, or becoming occurs through non-becoming, or existence comes into being because of non-existence, or that all things come about from emptiness.

The One Yang then moves and is seen dwelling in Heaven and the True.
一陽動處見天眞

    When Tai Ji begins to separate into Yin and Yang, the Yang moves and the Yin is still. There is then the separation of Heaven and Earth. The Yang moves towards Heaven and is seen dwelling there. This means it moves to the southerly direction and occupies the position of Qian (☰) in the Eight Diagrams and so becomes the symbol of the True (Reality).

When Yin unfolds, Yang is diminished, yet both tally in union.
陰舒陽慘相符合

    When the Yang is established in its proper position, Yin then extends itself out to hold the northerly position of Kun (☷). With Yin and Yang in their proper positions they then form a union in their interplay within the Ten Thousand Things.

The Nature of the Great Tao is unequaled in its depth.
大道參造化深

As the scripture on *Clarity and Tranquility of the Constant states,* "The Great Tao is without form, yet it gave birth to Heaven and Earth; the Great Tao is without impulse, yet it revolves and gives motion to the sun and moon; the Great Tao is without name, yet it eternally nourishes the Ten Thousand Things."

This is the Nature of the Great Tao, and there is nothing beyond it nor that which is deeper. Lao Zi then states, "I do not know its name, but if pressed to give it a name, I would call it Tao." Meaning, the term Tao is just an expedient term, as it has no real meaning, and because the depth of the Great Tao is so vast, because it is formless, because it has no impulse, it is then nameless.

In another text, the above verse reads:

"There was first chaos and the female principle [Yin]. Then the male principle [Yang] ascended and so Heaven was divided. The former [Yin] principle increased and the later [Yang] diminished, and both were able to then harmonize. Heaven and Earth then appeared, and the Great Reason [Tao], this then was Creation."

Xu Shenweng's Method for Preserving the Qi and Opening the Passes

徐神翁存氣開關法

Xu Sheng Wen Cun Qi Kai Guan Fa

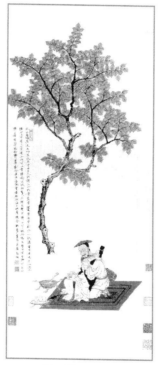

Xu Shenweng

Xu Shenweng, also called Xu Shouxin (守信), was born in Jiangshu province sometime during the Song dynasty (960–1279 CE).

Chen Tuan's Four Season Internal Kungfu

Cures

Cures false satiety [假盡飽, Jia Jin Bao], the abdomen is empty [腹虛, Fu Xu], but there is a feeling of fullness of Qi and breath [in it] [飽氣, Bao Qi].[75]

The main reason for this exercise and herbal formula is that some Taoist adepts who adhere to frequent and long meditation periods can, because of a feeling of fullness in the stomach and abdomen, a result of accumulating Qi, have no urge to eat (as can be experienced in fasting practices as well). Because of this, the seven orifices and functions within the body (see *The Passes*) are not being used and so may close, dysfunction, or become a barrier rather than a *pass* because of the lack of use. The exercise and herbal formula then keep these orifices and functions open and healthy, even if not being used.

Those who meditate frequently for long periods without eating should practice this exercise and take the herbal formula periodically because history has shown that many accomplished meditators have died from one form or another of gastric problems, either from intestinal, stomach, enteric, duodenal, celiac, abdominal, and ventral disorders. Many Asian cultivators also experience these problems from having spent years eating glutinous white rice every day, which overtime obstructs and clogs the

---

[75] Inability or fear to eat, yet feeling full and having no desire or appetite for eating. In Western medicine this is anorexia nervosa.

intestines, and if they don't adhere to a physical form of daily exercise to help remove this glutinous build up in the intestines, illness can occur.

Exercise

Sit in a fixed position. Use the two hands, crossing them over each other, and place them firmly on the shoulders. Then [with the head held still] gaze to the left. Mobilize the Qi in turning twelve mouthfuls.[76] Turn the eyes to the right and again inhale and exhale as before.

The Passes

The *Passes*, or *Barriers*, being referred to here are those connected to the ingestion and digestion processes of the body. Food properly passes through the following seven orifices when ingested to the final digestion and defecation processes:

1. *Kou* (口) the mouth, gateway to the lungs, and where food is first placed for ingestion.
2. *Ya* (牙) the teeth, the two leafs of the door, chews the food for ingestion.

---

[76] *Mobilizing the Qi* here means to visualize the Qi (like a thick cloud-like white substance) gathering in the mouth during twelve complete breaths. When turning the eyes from the left to the right side, swallow the gathered Qi in one gulp (嚥九息, Yan Jiu Xi, Ingesting Qi). After performing twelve complete breaths when gazing to the right, swallow the Qi/air in one gulp when turning to face front.

3. *Hou* (喉) the larynx or throat, the receptor of food being ingested.
4. *Shi Guan* (食管) the esophagus, the mouth of the stomach.
5. *Wei* (胃) the stomach or cardiac orifice connecting with the small intestine.
6. *Shi Er Zhi Chang* (十二指腸) the pyloric orifice (means "gate guard" in Latin), the duodenum. Literally means, "Twelve Sections of the Large Intestine."
7. *Gang Men* (肛門) the anus and its connection with the large intestine.

The *Nine Apertures*, also called Passes, are the two eye openings, two ear openings, two nostrils of the nose, mouth, urethra, and anus.

Verse on Death

The Heavenly Spirit [魂, Hun] leaves the body through the head, with the good person, into Heaven [天, Tian], and the Earthly Spirit [魄, Po] leaves by fundament[77] in the bad person, into the Earth [地, Di].

---

[77] The writer may have been injecting a little humor here, as *fundament* (臀, Tun) means the butt and buttocks, so the text is implying that the bad person departs this world from the butt. In the more serious Taoist perspective, it's said the bad person leaves through the bottom of the feet. When someone dies, a tradition is to feel the top of the head and the soles of the feet. Whichever area feels warm indicates whether the spirit went to a Heavenly realm via the head, or stayed on Earth (usually as a ghost) by passing through the feet.

Herbal Formula

Protecting Harmony Pills (保和丸, Bao He Wan)

Ingredients: 山查肉, Shan Zha Rou (二兩, Er Liang, 2 ounces); 神麴, Shen Qu (fried), 半夏, Ban Xia, 姜製汁, Jiang Zhi Zhi, and 茯苓, Fu Ling (各一兩, Ge Yi Liang, each one ounce); 羅茯子, Luo Fu Zi (炒, Chao, roasted and powdered), 陳皮, Chen Pi, and 連翹, Lian Qiao (各五錢, Ge Wu Qian, each five mace).

Preparation

First powder the Shen Qu and then form it into a paste by beating and mixing it together with the Shan Zha Rou, Ban Xia, Jiang Zhi Zhi, and Fu Ling. Next, add the Luo Fu Zi, Chen Pi, and Lian Qiao, and thoroughly mix them into a paste. Form the paste into 35 or more pills. Take one pill each day with a little [hot] soup or water.

The Verses Say (詩曰, Shi Yue)

Cook the lead in the night using the Jade Stove.
玉爐夜以烹鉛伏.

> During the hour of Zi (11:00 p.m. to 1:00 a.m.) sit in meditation concentrating on the lower abdomen (Jade Stove or Furnace) and develop heat that will simulate cooking the Jing (the Water element of the body), which here is more specifically referring to the saliva that has been ingested.

Seek Qian by regulating the Golden Cauldron.
金鼎時以治求乾.

> *Qian*, from the *Book of Changes,* means Heaven, or the creation aspect of nature. The *Golden Cauldron* is the brain where the Jing and Qi are transformed (into the Elixir, 丹, Dan), whereupon the Shen attaches itself to this newly formed elixir to create the Pill of Immortality (仙丸, Xian Wan).

The breath and Fire must not lack the 702.
息火不差七伯二.

> The *breath and Fire* here mean the heat of the Qi that has been mobilized. The number 702 (7+2=9) is an obscure term for acquiring the ability of revolving the Qi nine times through the Lesser Heavenly Circuit (小天周, Xiao Tian Zhou) over a hundred day period (伯, Ba), or as it is normally called, "One Hundred Days of Spiritual Work" (百日神功, Bai Ri Shen Gong).

Rumbling at the birth of awakening, the sound of thunder claps in the Muddy Pellet.
泥丸霹靂覺生寒.

> This verse is referring to an experience occurring within deep meditation states, where first the cultivator feels and hears a rumbling in the lower abdomen (the *birth of awakening*) that is followed by a loud internal sound, like thunder clapping

Medicinal Kung Regimes

within the brain (Muddy Pellet, Ni Wan Qi cavity). These two experiences signal that the cultivator has broken through the mundane mind into the spiritual consciousness, and so has entered into the immortal realms.

In Taoist Internal Alchemy writings, the phrase, "Hearing the sound of Thunder" is used quite often as a benchmark, in a manner of speaking, for the passage from mortality to immortality.

Appendix

Correlations and Positions of the Meridians According to the Eight Diagrams and Nine Palaces

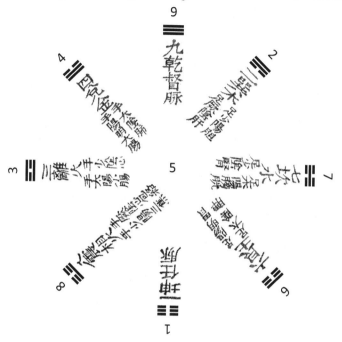

This image[78] and text are critical to understanding the relationships between the *Eight Diagrams*, *Nine Palaces* (the numbers associated with each trigram), the *Fourteen External Meridians,* and the *Six Zi* and *Six Qi*. Traditionally, this chart helped clarify the influences and characteristics of the meridians. Translations of the chart's text appear with the meridian illustrations. For those who wish to study these subjects more fully, please see *Book of Sun and Moon,* vol. I.

---

[78] From *A Collection on the Essentials of the Rivers He and Luo* (河洛精蘊, *He Lou Jing Yun),* four volumes, early Qing dynasty work (Reprinted by White Cloud Monastery, 1989.

9
Heaven ☰
(乾, Qian)

Control Meridian
(督脉, Du Mai)
28 points

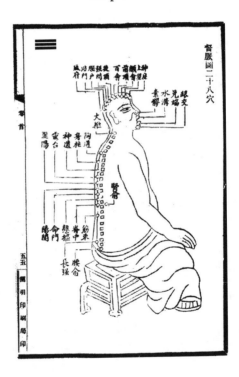

Appendix

4

Valley ☱
(兌, Dui)

Ultimate Yin Hand
(手太陰, Tai Yin)
Lung Meridian
(肺經, Fei Jing)
21 points

Metal
(金, Jin)

Bright Yang Hand
(手陽明, Shou Yang Ming)
Large Intestine Meridian
(大腸經, Da Chang Jing)
20 points

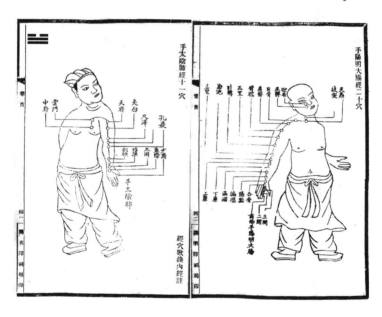

2

Wind ☴ (巽, Xun)　　　　**Wood** (木, Mu)

Faint Yin Foot　　　　**Young Yang Foot**
(足厥陰, Zu Jue Yin)　　(足少陽, Zu Shao Yang)
Liver Meridian　　　　**Gallbladder Meridian**
(肝經, Gan Jing),　　　　(膽經, Dan Jing)
25 points　　　　　　　　45 points

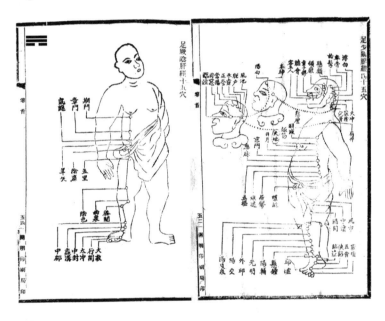

Appendix

3

Fire ☲ (離, Li)

Young Yin Hand
(手少陰, Shou Shao Yin)
Heart Meridian
(心經, Xin Jing)
9 points

Fire (火, Huo)

Ultimate Yang Hand
(手太陽, Tai Yang)
Small Intestine Meridian
(小腸經, Xiao Chang Jing)
19 points

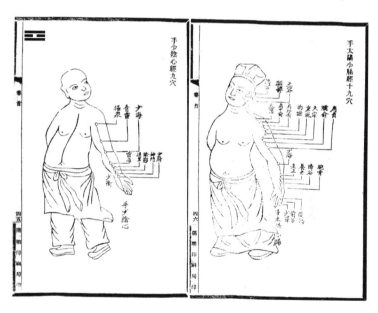

7

Water ☵
(坎, Kan)

Water
(水, Shui)

Young Yin Foot
(足少陰, Zu Shao Yin)
Kidney Meridian
(腎經, Shen Jing)
27 points

Ultimate Yang Foot
(足太陽, Zu Tai Yang)
Urinary Bladder Meridian
(膀胱經, Pang Guang Jing)
63 points

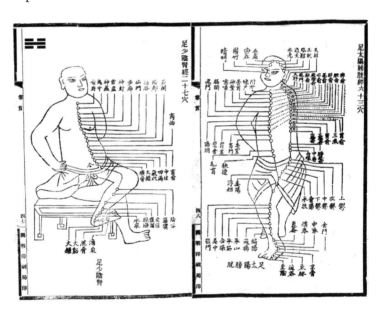

Appendix

8

Thunder ☳
(震, Zhen)

Secondary Fire
(相火, Xiang Huo).

Faint Yin Hand
(手厥陰, Shou Jue Yin)
Pericardium Meridian
(包絡經, Bao Luo Jing)
9 points

Young Yang Hand
(手少陽, Shou Shao Yang)
Triple Warmer Meridian
(三焦經, San Jiao Jing)
24 points

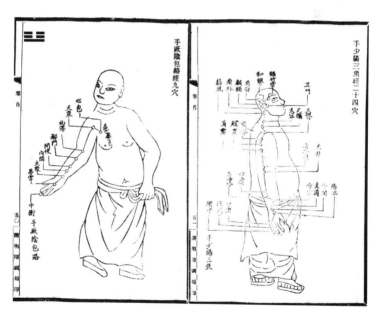

6

Mountain ☶	**Earth**
(艮, Gen)	(土, Tu)
Ultimate Yin Foot	**Bright Yang Foot**
(足太陰, Zu Tai Yin)	(足陽明, Zu Yang Ming)
Spleen Meridian	**Stomach Meridian**
(脾經, Pi Jing)	(胃經, Wei Jing)
22 points	45 points

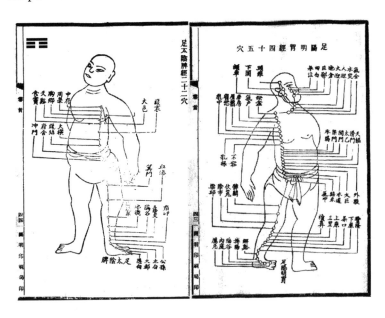

Appendix

1
Earth ☷
(坤, Kun)

Function Meridian
(任脉, Ren Mai)
24 points

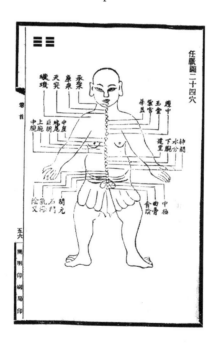

Twelve Earthly Branches

The Twelve Earthly Branches (十二地支, Shi Er Di Zhi)[79] are correlations to the months of a year and to the twelve two-hour periods of the day. These twelve divisions were originally calculated by Chinese astrologers observing the orbit of Jupiter, which they believed took twelve years to completely orbit the sun.[80] Thus, they were able to identify twelve months, twelve double-hours of the day, and even the 120 minutes within the double hour. The Earthly Branches also date back to the Shang dynasty, but originally they were not part of calendar calculation. This was solely done through the Ten Heavenly Stems, as it was the ritual calendar for the imperials of those times. When the astrological correlations began to gain popularity, however, the two systems came together to calculate the sixty-year

---

79 Like the term Stem (as in the *Ten Heavenly Stems*), "Branch" likewise relates to the branches of a plant or tree. Using these terms may seem confusing, but the idea is clearer if Stems are thought of as Celestial Stems, which connect to Heaven. Branches are termed Earthly Branches to imply the connection to Earth. Thus the two systems of calculation have to do with a human being's connection to Heaven and Earth, as shown with the Three Powers of Heaven, Humanity, and Earth.

80 Actually, it is 11.9 years to make a full orbit of the sun. Jupiter was held as a very auspicious star to the early Chinese, not only due to its enormous size, but because it was deemed as the protector of the Heavens. The star was named the "Year Star" because its orbit was used to calculate the years. Also because of its size, Jupiter was said to be the star where all the gods resided.

Appendix

cycles of time, a simple formula of 5 (Five Elements) x 12 (Earthly Branches).[81]

Twelve Earthly Branches	Twelve Hours	Twelve Astrological Animals	Twelve Months
子, Zi	11:00 p.m. to 1:00 a.m.	Rat (鼠, Shu)	11
丑, Chou	1:00 a.m. to 3:00 a.m.	Ox (牛, Niu)	12
寅, Yin	3:00 a.m. to 5:00 a.m.	Tiger (虎, Hu)	1
卯, Mao	5:00 a.m. to 7:00 a.m.	Rabbit (兔, Tu)	2
辰, Chen	7:00 a.m. to 9:00 a.m.	Dragon (龍, Long)	3
巳, Si	9:00 a.m. to 11:00 a.m.	Snake (蛇, She)	4
午, Wu	11:00 a.m. to 1:00 p.m.	Horse (馬, Ma)	5
未, Wei	1:00 p.m. to 3:00 p.m.	Goat (羊, Yang)	6
申, Shen	3:00 p.m. to 5:00 p.m.	Monkey (猴, Hou)	7
酉, You	5:00 p.m. to 7:00 p.m.	Rooster (雞, Ji)	8
戌, Xu	7:00 p.m. to 9:00 p.m.	Dog (狗, Gou)	9
亥, Hai	9:00 p.m. to 11:00 p.m.	Pig (猪, Zhu)	10

Chinese Hour Animal and Earthly Branch Correlations

Ultimate Yang Hours: Rat, Ox, Tiger, and Rabbit.
Young Yin Hours: Dragon and Snake.
Ultimate Yin Hours: Horse, Goat, Monkey, and Rooster.
Young Yang Hours: Dog and Pig.

Bright Yang and *Faint Yin* in this regard represent the appearance of the sun and moon. *Bright Yang* are all the daytime hours, and *Faint Yin* the nighttime hours.

---

[81] See *Book of Sun and Moon (I Ching)*, volumes I and II (Valley Spirit Arts, 2014).

Six Zi and Earthly Branch Correlations

The Six Zi term comes from the first ideogram of the Twelve Earthly Branches. *Zi* (子) represents the beginning of things as it is the first sign of the Twelve Earthly Branches, which have six Yang associations and six Yin ones. From this structure, we can see why each of the Four Seasons is divided into Six Zi—meaning 6 (Zi) x 4 (seasons) = 24 divisions of a year.

These types of calculations are clearly defined within the Six Zi, Six Qi, Twelve Meridians, and the *Twenty-Four Dao Yin Exercises*.[82]

Six Zi Calculations and Yi Jing Associations

The Six Zi are used in the *Book of Changes* when designating each line of a hexagram. The numerical value from the casting of each line determines which of the Six Zi terms apply, thereby designating the line as having either a Yin or Yang influence.

---

82 Ge Hong (葛洪) in his work *Master Who Embraces Simplicity* (抱朴子, *Bao Pu Zi*) explains that these six associations are not limited to just the idea of Six Zi. They are used in the six cyclical combinations of the *Six Ding* (丁) to show the six associations of when the energy of Heaven is storing (relating to the Six Yang Hand Meridians), or the six cyclical combinations of *Six Ji* (己) showing the six associations of when the Earth's energy is serving as a doorway (relating to the Six Yin Foot Meridians).

Appendix

The Six Zi, in regards to the classification of the individual lines in a six-line hexagram, were determined through the assigned numbers as used in stalk manipulation (9 & 6, 8 & 7, 5 & 4) when consulting the oracle *(Book of Changes)*. The names of the Six Zi relate to each of the six numbers used in casting a hexagram, just as they carry over into the naming of meridians, Qi energies, and so on.

Ultimate Yang and *Ultimate Yin* apply to changing Yang or Yin lines because these lines have reached their extreme position and so are changing from Yang to Yin or Yin to Yang, respectively, and given the numerical value of 9 *(Ultimate Yang)* and 6 *(Ultimate Yin)*.

A line is named *Young Yang* (7) when a single Yang line is positioned between two Yin lines in a trigram, and *Young Yin* (8) when a single Yin line appears between two Yang lines in a trigram—such as in the trigrams for Water ☵ *(Young Yang)* and Fire ☲ *(Young Yin)*.

Bright Yang (5) and *Faint Yin* (4) are determined when there is only one Yang or Yin line at the base of a trigram, such as with Thunder (☳) and Wind (☴).

Ultimate Yang and *Ultimate Yin* lines apply to trigrams with two Yang or Yin lines at the base, such as with Valley (☱) and Mountain (☶), and when all three lines of the trigrams are the same: Heaven (☰) and Earth (☷).

Chen Tuan's Four Season Internal Kungfu

Chart of the Five Forces Correlations

Yang
陽

Celestial:	**Green Dragon** Four-Clawed Azure Dragon	**Red Bird** Three-Legged Crow in the Sun
Terrestrial:	Earthly Dragons	Phoenix
Direction:	East	South
Element:	Wood	Fire
Activity:	Sprouting	Growth
Ten Stems: Interaction:	Shao Yang	Tai Yang
Yin-Yang:	True Yin	Yang
Yi Jing:	Brightness (Li) ☲ Sun	Creative (Qian) ☰ Heaven
Numbers:	3 and 8	2 and 7
Season:	Spring	Summer
Climate:	Wind	Heat
Planet:	Jupiter	Mars
Viscera:	Liver	Heart
Organ:	Eyes	Tongue
Fluids:	Tears	Sweat
Component:	Muscles/Sinews	Blood
Bowel:	Gallbladder	Small Intestine
Relation:	Father	Daughter
Spirit Name:	Dragon Mist	Red Ruler
Official Name:	Bright Container	Spirit Guard
Human Name:	Mang Zhang	Ling Guang
Attribute:	Perceptions	Impulses
Spirit Type:	Hun Spirit (Heavenly)	Human Spirit (Mortal)
Metallurgical:	Quicksilver	Cinnabar
Nei Dan:	True Mercury	PrimordialSpirit
Firing Tools:	Fuel	Furnace
Sexual:	Way of Yang (Penis)	Menstrual (Ovulation)

Appendix

Tai Ji 太極		Yin 陰	
Yellow Dragon	**White Tiger**		**Black Tortoise**
Five-Clawed Golden Dragon	*Jade Rabbit in the Moon*		*Snake and Tortoise/ Dark Warrior*
	White Crane		Two-Headed Deer
Center	West		North
Earth	Metal		Water
Maturity	Harvesting		Storage
10 Stems: Balanced Yin-Yang	Shao Yin		Tai Yin
Tai Ji	True Yang		Yin
Yin and Yang (– –) (—)	Abyss (Kan) ☵		Receptive (Kun) ☷
	Moon		Earth
5 and 10	4 and 9		1 and 6
Late/Long Summer	Autumn		Winter
Dampness	Dryness		Coldness
Saturn	Venus		Mercury
Spleen	Lungs		Kidneys
Mouth	Nose		Ears
Saliva	Mucus		Secretions
Flesh	Skin/Hair		Bones/Marrow
Stomach	large Intestine		Urinary Bladder
Ancestors	Mother		Son
	True Beauty		Water Spirit
	Complete Emptiness		Nourishing Infants
	Jian Bing		Zhi Ming
Consciousness	Feelings		Formations
Immortal Spirit (Original Spirit)	Po Spirit (Earthly/Animal)		Mind-Intent Spirit (Conscious Will)
Potable Gold	White Lead		Black Lead (Graphite)
Mind-Intent	True Lead		Primordial Essence
Cauldron	Bellows		Mixture
Embryo (Womb)	Way of Yin (Vagina)		Essence Seed (Semen/Sperm)

About the Translator

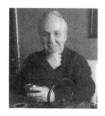

Stuart Alve Olson, longtime protégé of Master T.T. Liang (1900–2002), is a world renowned teacher, translator, and writer on Taoist philosophy, health, martial art, and internal arts. Since his early twenties, he has studied and practiced Taoism, Chinese Buddhism, and Asian related arts.

As of 2015, Stuart has published more than twenty books, many of which now appear in several foreign-language editions.

Biography

On Christmas Day, 1979, Stuart took Triple Refuge with Chan Master Hsuan Hua, receiving the disciple name Kuo Ao. In 1981, he participated in the meditation sessions and sutra lectures given by Dainin Katagiri Roshi at the Minnesota Center for Zen Meditation. In late 1981, he began living with Master T.T. Liang, studying Taijiquan, Taoism, Praying Mantis kung fu, and Chinese language under his tutelage.

In the spring of 1982 through 1984, Stuart undertook a two-year Buddhist bowing pilgrimage, "Nine Steps, One Bow." Traveling along state and county roads during the spring, summer, and autumn months, starting from the

Minnesota Zen Meditation Center in Minneapolis and ending at the border of Nebraska. During the winter months he stayed at Master Liang's home and bowed in his garage.

After Stuart's pilgrimage, he returned to Liang's home to continue studying with him. He and Master Liang then started traveling throughout the United States teaching Taijiquan to numerous groups, and continued to do so for nearly a decade.

In 1986, Stuart published his first four books on Taijiquan—*Wind Sweeps Away the Plum Blossoms, Cultivating the Ch'i, T'ai Chi Sword, Sabre & Staff,* and *Imagination Becomes Reality.*

In 1987, Stuart made his first of several trips to China, Taiwan, and Hong Kong. On subsequent trips, he studied massage in Taipei and taught Taijiquan in Taiwan and Hong Kong.

In 1989, he and Master Liang moved to Los Angeles, where Stuart studied Chinese language and continued his Taijiquan studies.

In early 1992, Stuart made his first trip to Indonesia, where he was able to briefly study with the kung fu and healing master Oei Kung Wei. He also taught Taijiquan there to many large groups.

In 1993, he organized the Institute of Internal Arts in St. Paul, Minnesota, and brought Master Liang back from California to teach there.

Appendix

In 2005, Stuart was prominently featured in the British Taijiquan documentary *Embracing the Tiger.*

In 2006, he formed Valley Spirit Arts with his longtime student Patrick Gross in Phoenix, Arizona.

In 2010, he began teaching for the Sanctuary of Tao and writing for its blog and newsletter.

In 2012, Stuart received the IMOS Journal Reader's Choice Award for "Best Author on Qigong."

Taoism Books

- *Actions & Retributions: A Taoist Treatise on Attaining Spiritual Virtue, Longevity, and Immortality,* Attributed to Lao Zi (Valley Spirit Arts, 2015).
- *Being Daoist: The Way of Drifting with the Current, Revised Edition* (Valley Spirit Arts, 2014).
- *Book of Sun and Moon (I Ching),* volumes I and II (Valley Spirit Arts, 2014).
- *Clarity & Tranquility: A Guide for Daoist Meditation* (Valley Spirit Arts, 2015).
- *Daoist Sexual Arts: A Guide for Attaining Health, Youthfulness, Vitality, and Awakening the Spirit* (Valley Spirit Arts, 2015).
- *Qigong Teachings of a Taoist Immortal: The Eight Essential Exercises of Master Li Ching-Yun* (Healing Arts Press, 2002).
- *Refining the Elixir: The Internal Alchemy Teachings of Taoist Immortal Zhang Sanfeng* (Valley Spirit Arts, 2016).

- *Tao of No Stress: Three Simple Paths* (Healing Arts Press, 2002).
- *Taoist Chanting & Recitation: At-Home Cultivator's Practice Guide* (Valley Spirit Arts, 2015).
- *The Immortal: True Accounts of the 250-Year-Old Man, Li Qingyun* by Yang Sen (Valley Spirit Arts, 2014).
- *The Jade Emperor's Mind Seal Classic: The Taoist Guide to Health, Longevity, and Immortality* (Inner Traditions, 2003).

Taijiquan Books

Chen Kung Series

- *Tai Ji Qi: Fundamentals of Qigong, Meditation, and Internal Alchemy*, vol. 1 (Valley Spirit Arts, 2013).
- *Tai Ji Jin: Discourses on Intrinsic Energies for Mastery of Self-Defense Skills*, vol. 2 (Valley Spirit Arts, 2013).
- *Tai Ji Tui Shou: Mastering the Eight Styles and Four Skills of Sensing Hands*, vol. 4 (Valley Spirit Arts, 2014).
- *Tai Ji Bing Shu: Discourses on the Taijiquan Weapon Arts of Sword, Saber, and Staff*, vol. 6 (Valley Spirit Arts, 2014).

   Forthcoming Books in Chen Kung Series

   - *Tai Ji Quan: Practice and Applications of the 105-Posture Solo Form*, vol. 3.
   - *Tai Ji San Shou & Da Lu: Mastering the Two-Person Application Skills*, vol. 5.

- *Tai Ji Wen: The Principles and Theories for Mastering Taijiquan*, vol. 7.
- *Imagination Becomes Reality: 150-Posture Taijiquan of Master T.T. Liang* (Valley Spirit Arts, 2011).
- *Steal My Art: The Life and Times of Tai Chi Master T.T. Liang* (North Atlantic Books, 2002).
- *T'ai Chi According to the I Ching—Embodying the Principles of the Book of Changes* (Healing Arts Press, 2002).
- *T'ai Chi for Kids: Move with the Animals,* illustrated by Gregory Crawford (Bear Cub Books, 2001).
- *Tai Ji Quan Treatise: Attributed to the Song Dynasty Daoist Priest Zhang Sanfeng,* Daoist Immortal Three Peaks Zhang Series (Valley Spirit Arts, 2011).
- *The Wind Sweeps Away the Plum Blossoms: Yang Style Taijiquan Staff and Spear Techniques* (Valley Spirit Arts, 2011).

Kung Fu Books

- *The Complete Guide to Northern Praying Mantis Kung Fu* (Blue Snake Books, 2010).
- *The Eighteen Lohan Skills: Traditional Shaolin Temple Kung Fu Training Methods* (Valley Spirit Arts, 2015).

CD and Downloadable Audio Recordings

- *Book of Tao and Virtue Contemplation Meditations* (CD and MP3 versions). Features Stuart Alve Olson's translation and narration of Lao Zi's *Tao De Jing* as it appears in the book *Taoist Chanting and Recitation.* The background music is by Deni Gendron, a longtime student of Stuart's. The two tracks comprise the *Book of Tao* (chapters 1 thru 37) and the *Book of Virtue* (chapters 38 thru 81). Each track can be used in separate meditation sessions that run about 40 minutes.

- *Setting Up the Foundation* (Instructional Recordings). Includes instructions on the different breathing techniques used for stimulating the Qi for completion of the Lesser Heavenly Circuit. Details on understanding the stages of Three in Front, Three on the Back; 36 and 24 Breaths; and Realizing the Dan Tian are given.

- *Yellow Court Scripture* (Course Recordings). The information in these 70 audio recordings is simply not attainable anywhere else. Recorded from online classes that Stuart conducted with a student over a year and a half, this commentary on the *Yellow Court Scripture* touches on Taoist philosophy, meditation, Internal Alchemy, medical Qigong, and the spirit world like no other Taoist material provides.

Appendix

DVDs

- **Chen Kung Series DVDs:** *Taiji Qigong, Taiji Sensing Hands,* and *Taiji Sword, Saber & Staff* (Valley Spirit Arts, 2013–15).
- *Eight Brocades Seated Qigong Exercises* (Valley Spirit Arts, 2012). Companion DVD to the book *Qigong Teachings of a Taoist Immortal.*
- *Healing Tigress Exercises* (Valley Spirit Arts, 2011).
- *Li Qingyun's Eight Brocades* (Valley Spirit Arts, 2014). Companion DVD to the book *The Immortal.*
- *Master T.T. Liang's 150-Posture Yang Style T'ai Chi Ch'uan Form* (Valley Spirit Arts, 2014).
- *Master T.T. Liang Taijiquan Demonstrations* (Valley Spirit Arts, 2014).
- *Tai Ji Quan Self-Defense Instructional Program* (3-DVD Set) (Valley Spirit Arts, 2011).
- *Tiger's Waist: Daoist Qigong Restoration* (Valley Spirit Arts, 2009).
- *Wind & Dew* (Valley Spirit Arts, 2012). This version of Wind & Dew was designed to work in conjunction with the Eight Brocades DVD (also the Li Qingyun version). All three DVDs also work with the teachings in the Setting Up the Foundation Audio Recordings.

Visit the Shop at Valley Spirit Arts for more information: www.valleyspiritarts.com/shop/

About the Publisher

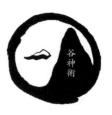

Valley Spirit Arts offers books and DVDs on Taoism, Taijiquan, and meditation practices primarily from author Stuart Alve Olson, longtime student of Master T.T. Liang and translator of many Taoist related works.

Its website provides teachings on meditation and Internal Alchemy, Taijiquan, Qigong, and Kung Fu through workshops, private and group classes, and online courses and consulting.

For more information as well as updates on Stuart Alve Olson's upcoming projects and events, please visit: www.valleyspiritarts.com.

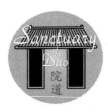

About the Sanctuary of Tao

The Sanctuary of Tao is a nonprofit organization dedicated to the sharing of Taoist philosophy and practices through online resources, yearly meditation retreats, and community educational programs. The underlying mission of the Sanctuary of Tao is to bring greater health, longevity, and contentment to its members and everyone it serves.

Please visit www.sanctuaryoftao.org for more information about the organization and its programs.

Made in the USA
Lexington, KY
06 June 2018